Integrating Health Humanities, Social Science, and Clinical Care

The health humanities are widely understood as a way to cultivate perspective, compassion, empathy, professional identity, and self-reflection among health professional students. This innovative book links humanities themes, social science domains, and clinical practice to invite self-discovery and recognition of universal human experiences.

Integrating Health Humanities, Social Science, and Clinical Care introduces critical topics that rarely receive sufficient attention in health professions education, such as cultivating resilience, witnessing suffering, overcoming unconscious bias, working with uncertainty, understanding professional and personal roles, and recognizing interdependence. The chapters encourage active engagement with a range of literary and artistic artifacts and guide the reader to question and explore the clinical skills that may be necessary to navigate clinical scenarios.

Accompanied by a range of pedagogical features including writing activities, discussion prompts, and tips for leading a health humanities seminar, this unique and accessible text is suitable for those studying the health professions, on both clinical and pre-clinical pathways.

Anna-leila Williams is Associate Professor of Medical Sciences at Quinnipiac University's Frank H. Netter MD School of Medicine.

Integrating Health Humanities, Social Science, and Clinical Care

A Guide to Self-Discovery, Compassion, and Well-being

ANNA-LEILA WILLIAMS

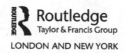

LONDON AND NEW YORK

First published 2019
by Routledge
2 Park Square, Milton Park, Abingdon, Oxon OX14 4RN

and by Routledge
52 Vanderbilt Avenue, New York, NY 10017

Routledge is an imprint of the Taylor & Francis Group, an informa business

British Library Cataloguing-in-Publication Data
A catalogue record for this book is available from the British Library

Library of Congress Cataloging-in-Publication Data
A catalog record has been requested for this book

ISBN: 978-1-138-30998-2 (hbk)
ISBN: 978-1-138-30999-9 (pbk)
ISBN: 978-1-315-14356-9 (ebk)

Typeset in Garamond
by Apex CoVantage, LLC

Visit the companion website: www.routledge.com/cw/williams

*To my mother, Lillian (Raya Hashim) Williams,
my sittoos, Mary (Waked Joseph) Raya Hashim and Ameena (Nasr)
Melhem Kesrouani [renamed Anna Williams by a United States
immigration officer], and all women of color whose experiences
as patients, caregivers, and healers have been ignored, denied, or
appropriated.*

CONTENTS

LIST OF ILLUSTRATIONS

PREFACE

I write today with the perspective of decades of clinical practice and a personal life redolent of the "full catastrophe" (Kabat-Zinn, 1990, p. 6). Questions about suffering, resilience, interdependence, uncertainty, meaning, and equity are central to the human experience; I have carried these questions throughout my adult life. While sitting with patients and families, I have witnessed people "live the questions" (Rilke, 2004, p. 27). And from time to time, in tiny, sacred moments, I glimpse an answer.

This book is an offering to health professionals and students who wrestle with questions about the human experience. It is also for those who have not encountered these questions yet. To stimulate the reader to self-discovery, I name insidious influences on health professionals, query the perceived norms of healthcare, and guide health professionals and students on a path to discover the myriad small moments that make life in clinical medicine precious.

May we all have courage and peace.

Anna-leila Williams
Hamden, Connecticut
Spring 2018

REFERENCE LIST

Kabat-Zinn, J. (1990). *Full catastrophe living: Using the wisdom of your body and mind to face stress, pain, and illness.* New York: Delacorte Press.

Rilke, M. R. (2004). *Letters to a young poet* (Rev. ed.). Translated by M. D. Herter Norton. New York and London: W. W. Norton & Company.

ACKNOWLEDGMENTS

Instructions for loving-kindness meditation, which appear in chapter 4, were published originally in the book, *Lovingkindness: The Revolutionary Art of Happiness*, 2002, Boston and London: Shambala, and are reprinted with permission from the author, Sharon Salzberg.

Some of the cancer family caregiver quotations that appear in chapter 7 were previously published in the *Journal of Palliative Medicine* (Williams, A., Bakitas, M. (2012). *Journal of Palliative Medicine*, 15(7), 775–783). The quotations are reprinted with permission from Mary Ann Liebert Publishing.

***

Many people helped this book come to fruition, some of whom I mention here and others I hold in my heart.

I am grateful to the Frank H. Netter MD School of Medicine administration for granting me sabbatical, and my colleagues who covered my responsibilities in my absence. I hope to have the opportunity to repay your munificence.

Special thanks to the wonderful teams at Routledge Publishing and Apex CoVantage who shepherded this book through editing, production, and marketing – I bow to your dedication and professionalism.

The librarians and library staff at Quinnipiac University, Yale University, and University College Cork deserve accolades for their diligence, kindness, and competence. I appreciate my inspirational and beautiful work spaces at Yale's Sterling Memorial Library and Divinity Library, and thank the maintenance and housekeeping workers who keep them so.

I deeply value the work of the intrepid souls who reviewed draft chapters: Will Bartlett, Christiane Nockels Fabbri, and Arthur Williams. Caitlin Glass reviewed the first draft of the entire book. Her insight, candor, and keen intellect improved the book immeasurably, and her friendship enriches my life.

I thank my students at Yale, Dartmouth, and Quinnipiac, who were the first audience for much of the material in this book. And I thank my teachers who opened my mind and heart to the human condition: Theresa Bergherr, Rita Charon, Roshi Joan Halifax, Frank Ostaseski, Rachel Naomi Remen, David Williams, and the venerable Thich Nhat Hanh.

My family offered boundless support and encouragement before and during this entire process. My late father, Ernest Nasib Williams, cultivated my passion for reading and education. He lived a life of faith, love, wit, and grit. My late mother, Lillian (Raya

Hashim) Williams was my model of perseverance and generosity. My late siblings, Theresa and Rechu, taught me to look for moments of delight, no matter the circumstance. My siblings, Arthur, David, and Mary Ann, fellow sojourners amid the full catastrophe, keep my feet on the ground and help me find humor even in the dark hours.

I am profoundly thankful to my husband, Will Bartlett, for his unflagging confidence, good cheer, magnificent music, and countless suppers. My son, David Nasib Bartlett, has been my writing companion, resident grammarian, and beacon during the times I wrote myself into a corner. Gratitude abounds.

1 INTRODUCTION: HEALTH HUMANITIES

PURPOSE OF THE BOOK

Health humanities is an emerging interdisciplinary field. Content is a synthesis of principles derived from the humanities *and* healthcare, not a superimposition of humanities on biomedicine (Jones, Wear, & Friedman, 2016). Health humanities curricula are recommended as a means of cultivating perspective, compassion, empathy, professional identity, and reflection among health professionals and health professional students (Garden, 2016; Shapiro, 2015). Many students welcome the opportunity to explore the wellspring of questions related to health humanities and refresh their inherent compassionate and empathic tendencies. However, throughout health professional education, biomedical sciences are valued so highly, it can be challenging to find a foray into health humanities.

More often than not, time devoted to health humanities curricula in the education of health professionals is undervalued (Bleakley, 2015a). I have heard health professions educators refer to humanities curricular content as "recess" – a respite from what they perceive to be the *real* curriculum. However, there is growing evidence to refute the exclusive domain of biomedical sciences as core curriculum. Social, behavioral, and environmental factors account for more than 50% of disease in the United States (Center for Disease Control and Prevention, 2014) and 25% of disease worldwide (Blas & Kurup, 2010). The staggering influence of social, behavioral, and environmental factors on disease development make the integration of behavioral and social science content into health professions curriculum indisputable and indispensable if we truly intend to improve the health of the population. With a behavioral and social science lens, we may be able to address health disparities and inequities, social determinants of health, cultural awareness, and social accountability. In the same vein, health humanities, with emphasis on first person narrative for patients, family members, and health professionals, help us understand and appreciate the social, cultural, and spiritual influences on illness, which when ignored, can tragically impede the effectiveness of biomedicine.

The purpose of this book is to present a practical guide for a health humanities–social science curriculum that makes overt links to clinical care and emphasizes self-discovery and self-awareness. By unambiguously tying health humanities and social science to clinical practice, learners are encouraged to question and explore the clinical skills necessary to navigate a clinical scenario. At the end of each chapter, I recommend literary and artistic artifacts that integrate with clinical science curricula, thus reinforcing relevance to the practice of medicine. The recommended artifacts use a variety of media, such as written word, spoken word, photography, and videography, to express their content and will likely have broad aesthetic appeal. For example, learners who are not attracted to literature will find visually mediated artifacts elsewhere in the book, and similarly, those who do not respond to visual images will be sated by the literary pieces. Writing prompts provided throughout the book assure learners have the opportunity for reflection on their perspectives of patients, healthcare workers, and the healthcare system.

The book emphasizes the value of self-discovery and self-awareness. In a healthcare arena dominated by technology and fueled by economic outcomes, it is easy for us, as health professionals, to drift from our calling to serve fellow human beings and lose awareness of our untoward effect on patients and colleagues (Churchill, 2003). When we are self-aware, we are less likely to engage in aberrant and unprofessional behavior that threatens our own well-being, as well as that of our patients and colleagues. Moreover, self-awareness is a necessary condition for health professionals to engage in authentic, compassionate relationships with co-workers and those in our care.

OVERVIEW OF HEALTH HUMANITIES

The fields of healthcare and humanities are distinct, and until relatively recently, their canons had little overlap. Yet, when we focus on content, it is easy to welcome the marriage of the two fields. Both healthcare and humanities are committed to exploring what it means to be human, in all the manifestations of our species – biological, psychological, social, and spiritual. The fundamental differences between the two fields derive from their ways of knowing, and the privilege given to reductive versus experiential knowledge (Boudreau & Fuks, 2014). Eric R. Kandel, MD (2012, p. 449), Columbia University professor of neuroscience, Director of the Kavli Institute for Brain Science, and Nobel laureate writes:

> Artists and scientists alike are reductionists, but they have different ways of knowing and making sense of the world. Scientists make models of elementary features of the world that can be tested and reformulated. These tests rely on removing the subjective biases of the observer and relying on objective measurements or evaluations. Artists also form models of the world, but rather than being empirical approximations, artists create subjective impressions of the ambiguous reality they encounter in their everyday lives.

Humanities scholarship, illness experiences, and clinical practice are driven by questions about suffering, resilience, hope, and meaning. They have informed each other for centuries and in the near past have given birth to the unique discipline of health humanities (Dolan, 2015). Our pathways to knowledge and ways of knowing expand when we recognize and embrace the synergy of mind, heart, and body. With new ways of knowing, we respect our experiences, nourish our human capacity for insight, and enhance our clinical skills and acumen (Chiavaroli, 2017).

As with any nascent field of study, the boundaries that define health humanities are permeable with a tendency toward inclusion. That said, prevailing consensus at present implies the health humanities canon encompasses stories of illness, disability, and caring, presented by historians, social scientists, ethicists, and artists, as well as patients, healthcare workers, and family members (Bleakley, 2015b). The stories may be expressed through multiple media, including visual art, theater, music, written word, and spoken word. The emergent state of the health humanities is both strength and weakness. Its strength springs from the dynamic creativity that accompanies boundlessness and the expansion of thought that is inherent in diversity. The weakness stems from its lack of cohesion. Critics who want to cull health humanities from biomedical education need only point to an unsubstantiated corner of the field to undermine the entire discipline. During this early period, while scholarship, metrics, and efficacy studies are in development, health humanities remain vulnerable to the whims of the dominant biomedical culture.

PHILOSOPHICAL UNDERPINNINGS

Underpinning this text are basic tenets of philosophy of medicine. Although one can certainly navigate this book, and even clinical practice, without any understanding of philosophy, a brief orientation to the basic tenets may add depth to one's experiential learning.

Philosophy of Medicine is a growing field with emerging work devoted to understanding disease causation, characterizing notions of health and disease in different social contexts, illustrating the genesis of mental illness stigmatization, and more (Carel & Cooper, 2014). Here I focus exclusively on phenomenology – the philosophical study of perceived human experience.

PHENOMENOLOGY

It is essential that health professionals understand our patients' experiences of illness. The more we are able to comprehend, the more likely we are to come up with an accurate diagnosis, and develop and execute a treatment plan that aligns with the patient's values and life. Anything short of that is an exercise in futility for the health professional and a danger to the patient. One important way of understanding the patient's experience of illness is through his or her first-person narrative, which philosophers of medicine refer to as phenomenology. Phenomenological approaches give us the patient's view of the life changing and disorienting aspects of illness, and explore what it is like to instill bodily dysfunction into one's everyday life (Carel, 2008; Carel, 2011; Svenaeus, 2000; Toombs, 1988). The literary and artistic artifacts recommended in this book are primarily phenomenological, with patients sharing their lived experience with illness and suffering.

CONCEPTUAL FRAMEWORKS

Conceptual frameworks provide a systematic approach to organizing key variables for a scholarly undertaking and promote a common language (Maxwell, 2013). Constructed from the extant literature, a conceptual framework makes one's assumptions, expectations, beliefs, and theories transparent, and displays purported interactions and relationships among variables, thus providing the argument for the relevance of one's scholarship and the methods used to define it (Ravitch & Riggan, 2012). For this text, three conceptual frameworks that build on each other helped inform the inquiries made into the human experience, as well as the selection of literary and artistic artifacts.

THE BIOPSYCHOSOCIAL MODEL OF MEDICINE

First proposed in the 1970s by physician and University of Rochester School of Medicine professor, George Engel, MD, the Biopsychosocial Model of Medicine was radical for its time, taking a firm stance in opposition to the "reductionistic," "physicalistic," "dualistic" biomedical model. Dr. Engel (1977, p. 132) wrote,

> the existing biomedical model does not suffice. To provide a basis for understanding the determinants of disease and arriving at rational treatments and patterns of health care, a medical model must also take into account the patient, the social context in which he lives, and the complementary system devised by society to deal with the disruptive effects of illness, that is, the physician role and the health care system. This requires a biopsychosocial model.

Engel's Biopsychosocial Model of Medicine offers a practical framework to explore suffering, disease, and illness from the patient's experience. By moving beyond the biological confines to also attend to the patient's psychological, social, and cultural context of illness, the health professional can be responsive to patients with dysphoria and dysfunction, regardless of the origin of the symptoms.

EXPLANATORY MODEL OF DISEASE

Arthur Kleinman, MD, MS, physician and anthropologist, was able to use the centrality of the patient experience to articulate new understanding of disease and illness. Dr. Kleinman's (1988) Explanatory Model of Disease takes a holistic view of illness and its impact on individuals and families. Dr. Kleinman posits that each person's illness is distinct, characterized by an individual's culture and history. Although similar to the Biopsychosocial Model, the Explanatory Model is emphasizes the stimulus of culture on one's interpretation of symptoms and recognition of the influence of family and social structure on one's approach to treatment.

Kleinman, Eisenberg, and Good (1978, p. 258) define illness as "experiences of disvalued changes in states of being and in social function; the human experience of sickness." This definition is in contrast to disease, which the authors define as "abnormalities in the structure and function of body organs and systems." When we consider that health professionals exist to care for patients, and that the word patient comes from Latin roots meaning one who suffers, it seems rational that we concern ourselves at least as much with illness as with disease. Although some health professions have chosen to discard the word patient in favor of perceived egalitarian, non-hierarchical language such as client or health consumer, I assert that someone who is ill is at risk of suffering. In this book, I will use the word patient, which remains the primary reference label used at medical, physician assistant, and nursing schools in the United States.

SOCIAL ECOLOGICAL MODEL OF HEALTH

The Social Ecological Model of Health was developed as a collaborative effort of the World Health Organization to help prioritize equity and recognize illness and health within the socioeconomic and occupational context of an individual's life. The model acknowledges global differences in perceptions, challenges, and opportunities related to health while considering the psychosocial, economic, educational, cultural, and environmental conditions in which people live, work, worship, and engage in leisure activities (Dahlgren & Whitehead, 1991). The model categorizes illness and health as consequences of political and social agendas, with disenfranchised and vulnerable members of the population at risk for exploitation. With the individual at the center of the model, the display includes lifestyle behaviors, and community and social networks, and shows the pressures exerted by agriculture and food production, education, work environment, unemployment, water and sanitation, healthcare services, and housing. The Social Ecological Model of Health highlights the many ways and venues that affect an individual's health.

THE MODELS IN THIS BOOK

Throughout this book I periodically revisit the three conceptual frameworks (Biopsychosocial Model, Explanatory Model of Disease, and Social Ecological Model of Health), with the aim to explicate principle ideas. The models underscore the complex interplay among health, illness, disease, and suffering, and help assure that discussions and examples in this book are multidimensional representations of the human experience.

ILLNESS LANGUAGE AND NARRATIVES

Linguists, sociologists, anthropologists, and others have explored extensively the language of illness, and the effect language has on the person expressing the words and the person receiving the words. By extension, illness language comprises illness narrative. The language-narrative connection leads us to two questions: What effect does language have on the story, and what effect does the story in turn have on us – especially on our perceptions of health and illness? In this introductory chapter, I briefly highlight some of the formative work in the fields of illness language and illness narrative to heighten the reader's awareness of the subtleties of language that one may encounter later in the book. In addition, attention to language can be a venture toward self-discovery when one reads one's own written reflections as suggested during the activities at the end of each chapter.

LANGUAGE

Let's think for a moment about the English language words often used in association with illness stories. Perhaps you have heard people say someone is "battling cancer," "putting up a good fight," while someone else is "controlling her hypertension" while helping her father who "suffers from Alzheimer's" and her daughter who is "down" with the flu. Furthermore, nations have "eradicated" small pox and "wiped out" polio. Each of these phrases characterizes illness and disease as fierce and formidable opponents that must be handled aggressively. Linguist Suzanne Fleischman (1999) explores the psychological substrate from which illness language emerges and the unconscious meta-message the language conveys. Her thoughtful, scholarly reflection compares the language of physicians and patients, and the language transitions that occur, especially for patients, as disease becomes part of their self-identity. Fleischman, and Susan Sontag (1978) before her, argue that by using aggressive metaphorical language, we mythologize and objectify disease. The objectification helps us consider disease as something that we overcome and expunge, like a military conquest, rather than something that is integral to our lives. Within the linguistic paradigm, the patient – the one who suffers – is either a warrior who is up to the disease challenge, or a victim who is not.

Other scholars have looked at sociolinguistic variations in illness language usage by gender, age, socioeconomic classification, and disease type. Using sophisticated methodologies and analytic techniques, Charteris-Black and Seale (2010) in their book, *Gender and the Language of Illness*, describe language differences among different subpopulations of British residents. For example, the men in their study consistently used language that distanced themselves from their illness and allowed them to avoid talking about their illness. They termed this language strategy *reification*, which means, "treating either the ailing body or psycho-emotional responses to the ailing body as material entities rather than as part of a lived experience" (p. 56). Men were 50% more likely to refer to their illness as a "problem" or "difficulty" than women were. The traditional masculine discursive style allows the patient to

> view themselves from an external viewpoint, considering their bodies as things to be examined from the outside, in much the same way as they might face problems in the material world such as fixing a faulty tap or a leaking roof. The reification involved in this suggests that these men may be distancing themselves from inner states related to their illness conditions.
>
> (p. 59)

Charteris-Black and Seale characterize traditional feminine discursive style as transformational language, which uses elements of self-reflection about the illness and proactive agency in response to the illness. In their study, women were significantly more likely than men were to use cognitive and affective verbs such as "think," "know," and "need." The authors state, "we have seen how women engage more fully with the experience – either tentatively by expressing their uncertainties about illness or less tentatively by clearly stating their needs and desires" (p. 118).

Of interest, some linguistic gender differences blur when the authors controlled for socioeconomic classification. For example, men in high socioeconomic groups and women in low socioeconomic groups were similar in their use of emotionally expressive adjectives related to their illness experience. There appears to be a generational difference among men, with younger men adopting a more traditional feminine discursive style, especially when talking about feelings. A generational divide is also apparent among women, with older women adopting an authoritative language style related to illness discourse that other demographic groups do not demonstrate.

We still have much to learn about illness language and its implications. Global and cross-cultural exploration of illness language will likely provide rich insights into the human experience of illness.

ILLNESS NARRATIVES

Using the Biopsychosocial Model of Medicine (Engel, 1977) and the Explanatory Model of Disease (Kleinman, 1988) as our conceptual frameworks, we know illness is unique to the individual. In turn, each illness narrative is also unique. That said, illness narratives are predicated on the larger culture and cultural beliefs (Frank, 2010). Medical anthropologists have shared insights about illness from cultures around the world. As an example, we will look at one of the dominant sociocultural illness stories in the United States from the perspective of patients and health professionals.

PATIENTS

In the United States, one of the dominant sociocultural illness stories, especially with a life-altering diagnosis, pits the patient-warrior against the disease-perpetrator in a combat story. How does the combat story unfold? To begin, the story draws a rigid boundary between those who are ill and those who are healthy, those who are part of the battle and those who are not. On many occasions, I have heard patients in the chemotherapy center say – with a mix of awe and terror – something like, "There's a whole world here that I never knew existed before." Patients must quickly learn to navigate the new world, with scant access to guides or training. Physician, Columbia University professor, and author Rita Charon, MD, PhD (2006, p. 21) writes in *Narrative Medicine: Honoring the Stories of Illness*,

> Unlike other divides – gender, race, class, place, age, time – that separate one human being from another, the divide between the sick and well is capricious, unpredictable, sometimes reversible but in the end irrevocable. It spares no one. . . . The world is transformed after the diagnosis of a serious disease, not only in the corporeal aspects of everyday life – now with pain, now with pills, now with slippers, now with a wheelchair – but in the deepest wells of meaning – now with limits, regrets, forced separations, final plans.

Having stepped into the new world of disease, patients relinquish their privacy and in some measure their dignity, and place their faith in a cadre of health professionals. Drawing on military rhetoric, the patient's disease is inimical and often insidious, working at a cellular level to destroy them. In this sociocultural illness story, there is no opportunity for negotiation with the disease-perpetrator. The only option for the patient is to put on the armor and fight. But here's the catch – the vast majority of the patient's most potent weapons are inaccessible to them. Healthcare workers must wield the weapons, in the form of therapeutics, on behalf of the patient, thus rendering the patient a passive warrior whose body is the battlefield. What can patients do in this world? They can arrive on time, follow directions precisely, show appreciation and gratitude, pay the bills, and fight. What does fight mean in this context? The weapons in the patient's personal arsenal include their will to live, their social network, their positive attitude, and prayer. And with this, they are judged by society writ large as to how well they assume the role of warrior. It is frequently a freighted circumstance for patients.

Like every warrior, there comes a time when the patient is battle weary. One young mother, while receiving chemotherapy for non-small cell carcinoma of the lung, told me that she yearns to return to simpler times. She said, "I want to kick back and dangle my toes in the water without a care for blood cell counts and ejection fractions." However, the carefree times remain elusive to most once they receive their diagnosis and are ushered into the new world of disease. The psychological and emotional separation imposed by our sociocultural illness narrative contributes to their sense of alienation, loneliness, and grief, all of which erode their personal arsenal (Sontag, 1978). It is nearly impossible for someone to bolster their will to live and their positive attitude when they are alienated from their social support system, whose members still live in the world of the healthy. Author Nancy Riggs (2017, p. 121) shares her feelings of estrangement while undergoing chemotherapy for breast cancer,

> In treatment, the wrongness I feel in my life is a wrongness reflected in my body – my steroid puffy face, my bald head, my lopsided chest. And spending my days at the cancer center: It's something I'm part of. I make sense there somehow. A lot more sense than I make at the gym or the elementary school or the grocery store or work meetings – or all the other places I've sat outside of for too long in my car taking deep breaths as I attempt to return to civilian life.

This is where health professionals may be helpful. As health professionals, we traverse the boundary between the world of the healthy and the world of the ill on a regular basis. There may even come a point when the boundary between health and illness blurs and the aggressive, disease-battle metaphor of the sociocultural illness narrative no longer applies. A new story calls to us, one that offers health professionals, patients, and families the opportunity for meaning making and relationship building.

Throughout this book you will have the opportunity to consider new and familiar stories that call to you.

HEALTH PROFESSIONALS

We have talked about the alienating effect the sociocultural illness narrative can have on patients. Now let's think about what effect the combat story might have on health professionals. What is it like, day after day, year after year, to be "in the trenches" – "battling disease"? Is the battle narrative sustainable over a career? Does one need to believe the battle narrative to be an effective clinician? Whom does the battle narrative support? Does the battle narrative influence how we interact with patients, colleagues, and our family and friends?

I assert the battle narrative could be a major contributor to burnout among health professionals. By extension, I further assert the battle narrative may contribute to elevated levels of depression, chemical substance use, and suicide experienced by some of the health professions (see chapter 5 Resilience and Burnout). Many of us are called to be health professionals by a deep inner drive to serve and care for our fellow human beings. Then, we quickly find ourselves with key roles in an illness narrative that casts us as weapons purveyors in a battle against disease. Working within this sociocultural illness narrative, our attention shifts from patient to disease, and our actions shift from caring to combat. When we are no longer responding to our call to service, it becomes difficult to find meaning in our work. With the absence of meaningful work, we are vulnerable to burnout, depression, and self-medication with alcohol and other readily available drugs (see chapter 5 Resilience and Burnout). However, this is not a path of inevitability.

We all know health professionals who live authentic lives and have meaningful careers of service and caring. What is their illness narrative? How do they keep the din of the dominant sociocultural illness battle narrative in abeyance? These are important research questions that need to be studied in our pursuit to mitigate burnout, depression, chemical substance use, and suicide among health professionals. While we wait for those research results (or conduct the research ourselves), we can aim to have a handle on our own illness narrative. If we continually renew our commitment to our calling, then we will be able to realize rapidly when we have drifted from our narrative. With self-awareness, we can decide if we are ready for a new story or if we need to reorient to our original path of service and caring.

I invite you to bring to mind the stories that inform your life, especially as they relate to health and illness. For example, consider childhood stories you heard that contextualized illness among your family members or for yourself. Was illness believed to be a curse, the result of receiving the "evil eye"? Was the sick person thought to be a victim or somehow personally deficient or responsible for their ailment? What stories did you hear about caregivers? Notice how these stories might influence your behavior, interpretation of experiences, and distillation of meaning. Throughout this book, I encourage you to revisit the dominant sociocultural illness narrative, as well as your personal illness narrative, to see which supports meaning making and relationship building as we explore the experience of being human.

CLOSING – WHAT YOU CAN EXPECT

Each of the subsequent chapters in this book presents a key theme about the human experience that is especially relevant to clinical care. My aim is to discuss the theme from multiple perspectives, and when possible, to prioritize the perspectives of patients, family members, and health professionals. I draw from the behavioral and social sciences literature, and the expertise of philosophers, historians, and theologians. The content directly relates to clinical care and the health professional. At the start of each chapter, I provide an *Integration Note* that includes recommendations for how chapter content may integrate with clinical science curricula.

I close each chapter with suggested activities to help the reader internalize and personally experience some of the themes discussed. The activities include exploration of a literary or artistic artifact, and the invitation to respond to a writing prompt. The writing prompt is designed to promote the learner's reflection and self-discovery. I provide learning objectives for the activities. For faculty, I have created guides to facilitate the activities. The guides can be found in Appendices A and B.

The reader may use the chapters out of order and independent of each other; however, most chapters will directly or indirectly reference the foundational material presented in this introductory chapter.

REFERENCE LIST

Blas, E., & Kurup, A. S. (Eds.). (2010). *Equity, social determinants, and public health programmes.* World Health Organization. Retrieved from http://apps.who.int/iris/bitstream/handle/10665/44289/9789241563970_eng.pdf;jsessionid=1C2FBBCB9E90C73A898E12D88FE9D8F0?sequence=1

Bleakley, A. (2015a). When I say medical humanities in medical education. *Medical Education, 49,* 959–960.

Bleakley, A. (2015b). *Medical humanities and medical education: How the medical humanities can shape better doctors.* London and New York: Routledge, Taylor & Francis.

Boudreau, J. D., & Fuks, A. (2014). The humanities in medical education: Ways of knowing, doing and being. *Journal of Medical Humanities, 36*(4), 321–336.

Carel, H. (2008). *Illness: The cry of the flesh.* Stocksfield, UK: Acumen.

Carel, H. (2011). Phenomenology and its application in medicine. *Theoretical Medicine and Bioethics, 32,* 33–46.

Carel, H., & Cooper, R. (Eds.). (2014). *Health, illness, and disease: Philosophical essays.* London and New York: Routledge, Taylor & Francis.

Center for Disease Control and Prevention. (2014). *What are determinants of health and how are they related to social determinants of health.* Author. Retrieved from www.cdc.gov/nchhstp/socialdeterminants/faq.html

Charon, R. (2006). *Narrative medicine: Honoring the stories of illness*. New York: Oxford University Press.

Charteris-Black, J., & Seale, C. (2010). *Gender and the language of illness*. London: Palgrave Macmillan.

Chiavaroli, N. (2017). Knowing how we know: An epistemological rationale for the medical humanities. *Medical Education, 51*, 13–21.

Churchill, L. R. (2003). Teaching professional ethics in an environment of medical commercialism. In R. A. Carson, C. R. Burns, & T. R. Cole (Eds.), *Practicing the medical humanities: Engaging the physician and patient* (pp. 7–24). Hagerstown, MD: University Publishing.

Dahlgren, G., & Whitehead, M. (1991). *Policies and strategies to promote social equity in health*. Stockholm: Institute for Future Studies. Retrieved from https://core.ac.uk/download/pdf/6472456.pdf

Dolan, B. (Ed.). (2015). *Humanitas: Readings in the development of the medical humanities*. San Francisco, CA: University of California Medical Humanities.

Engel, G. L. (1977). The need for a new medical model: A challenge for biomedicine. *Science, 196*(4286), 130.

Fleischman, S. (1999). I am, I have, I suffer from. . . : A linguist reflects on the language of illness and disease. *Journal of Medical Humanities, 20*(1), 3–32.

Frank, A. W. (2010). *Letting stories breathe: A socio-narratology*. Chicago, IL: University of Chicago Press.

Garden, R. (2016). Social studies: The humanities, narrative, and the social context of the patient-professional relationship. In T. Jones, D. Wear, & L. D. Friedman (Eds.), *Health humanities reader* (pp. 127–137). New Brunswick, NJ: Rutgers University.

Jones, T., Wear, D., & Friedman, L. D. (2016). The why, the what, and the how of the medical/health humanities. In T. Jones, D. Wear, & L. D. Friedman (Eds.), *Health humanities reader* (pp. 1–11). New Brunswick, NJ: Rutgers University.

Kandel, E. R. (2012). *The age of insight: The quest to understand the unconscious in art, mind, and brain, from Vienna 1900 to the present*. New York: Random House.

Kleinman, A. (1988). *The illness narratives: Suffering, healing, and the human condition*. New York: Basic Books.

Kleinman, A., Eisenberg, L., & Good, B. (1978). Culture, illness, and care: Clinical lessons from anthropologic and cross-cultural research. *Annals of Internal Medicine, 88*, 251.

Maxwell, J. A. (2013). *Qualitative research design: An interactive approach* (3rd ed.). Thousand Oaks, CA: Sage.

Ravitch, S. M., & Riggan, M. (2012). *Reason and rigor: How conceptual frameworks guide research*. Thousand Oaks, CA: Sage.

Riggs, N. (2017). *Bright hour: A memoir of living and dying*. New York: Simon and Schuster.

Shapiro, J. (2015). Health humanities and its satisfactions. In B. Dolan (Ed.), *Humanitas: Readings in the development of the medical humanities*. San Francisco, CA: University of California Medical Humanities.

Sontag, S. (1978). *Illness as metaphor*. New York: Farrar, Straus, Giroux.

Svenaeus, F. (2000). The body uncanny – further steps toward a phenomenology of illness. *Medicine, Health Care and Philosophy, 3*, 125–137.

Toombs, S. K. (1988). Illness and the paradigm of lived body. *Theoretical Medicine, 9*(2), 201–226.

2 PATIENT AS STORYTELLER: DETERMINANTS OF HEALTH

INTRODUCTION

Patients come to us with their stories. In all healthcare scenarios, other than medical emergencies, the encounter involves the patient (or surrogate) telling a story of bodily and/or psychological function gone awry, being maintained, or improving. The stories range from perfunctory to profound, somber to sublime, humorous to tragic – and more often than not, are a complicated montage of all of the above. The patient, as storyteller, knows the story best. Harvard University psychology professor Daniel Gilbert, PhD (2007, p. 66) writes,

> If we want to know how a person feels, we must begin by acknowledging the fact that there is one and only one observer stationed at the critical point of view . . . she is the only person who has even the slightest chance of describing "the view from in here," which is why her claims serve as the gold standard against which all other measures are measured.

With this passage Professor Gilbert identifies the patient as the one with the ideal vantage point, the most dense and nuanced perspective of the encounter with illness. When we believe our patients to be master storytellers, we have the opportunity to understand the impact of illness on the totality of their life: work, family, sexuality, sorrow, sense of vulnerability, creativity, aspirations – the interwoven tangle that makes up human life.

This chapter looks at the value and challenge of recognizing the patient as storyteller. To that end, I compare the processes of *taking* a patient history and *receiving* a patient history. I present social determinants of health as major drivers of disease and consider the privilege afforded health professionals who understand patients' social and physical environment. I describe the different types of illness stories patients tell, and then explore the effect of patients' stories on the health professional. Finally, I present data on recent efforts to amplify patients' voices and the influence patient input is having on the healthcare industry. The chapter concludes with activities to help the reader experience the patient as storyteller and engage with the material.

HISTORY TAKING COMPARED TO HISTORY RECEIVING

The first step in nearly every clinical encounter is to elicit the patient's story. As the health professional queries and listens, in addition to establishing rapport and demonstrating respect and concern, he or she engages in vital data gathering that contributes to proper diagnosis, treatment, and prevention. The precise skills involved in healthcare communication are both a science and an art – and are beyond the scope of this chapter. Instead, I invite the reader to consider how, as health professionals, we orient ourselves to take the patient's history or receive the patient's history.

HISTORY TAKING

In clinical practice, you have likely heard the phrase "take a history." This is, at present, the common jargon of health professionals. History taking roughly aligns with the clinician-centered interview, which means it is a fact-gathering endeavor. The health professional pursues a precise line of inquiry with the goal of *taking* information from the patient. It is clinician-driven, reductionistic, often algorithmic, and purported to be efficient. In this age of electronic health records, taking a patient history, in many circumstances, is relegated to checkboxes and dropdown menus. The highly structured format of history taking keeps health professional and patient seemingly on task. Which raises the question: What precisely is the task at hand? There are health professionals who believe the task is to discern the source of the patient's discomfort and provide proper treatment. For other health professionals, the clinical encounter is purely a transactional relationship. There are also many health professionals who believe the encounter is a combination of patient-directed service and transaction. In *The Illness Narratives: Suffering, Healing, and the Human Condition*, Arthur Kleinman, MD (1988, p. 253) posits, "The purpose of medicine is both control of disease processes and care for the illness experience." If you agree with Dr. Kleinman, then history taking is inadequate and inefficient for the task. By design, history taking directs the health professional to circumnavigate details of the patient's life that can help to understand the patient's malady and the means by which the patient will execute the requisite treatment plans. In the next section, we look at a sample patient case to show some of the limitations of history taking.

PATIENT CASE

Your patient is a healthy young man with new onset non-productive cough and chest tightness. In a matter of minutes you ask the questions to determine that he does not smoke and his symptoms are unlikely to be infectious or cardiac in origin. A quick physical exam confirms your suspected diagnosis of reactive airway disease. You give the patient a prescription based on current evidence-based standards for treatment and move on, satisfied that you made the correct diagnosis and prescribed appropriate treatment. In this scenario, history taking seems like part of an efficient process. However, even in this simple case of an acute illness in a normally healthy young person, disease resolution may be stymied if the patient has challenges elsewhere in his social ecology. If he is unable to adhere to his treatment plan, he can develop an exacerbation of his symptoms which will lead to his return to the healthcare system – thereby rendering the process highly *in*efficient. This particular young man recently left a violent relationship and has come upon hard economic times. He is living with friends. He is sleeping on an old couch permeated with dust. Two of the people he lives with smoke cigarettes. This means that he has ongoing exposure to environmental triggers for reactive airway disease: dust and cigarette smoke. When the young man arrives at the pharmacy to pick up the prescription, the price for the medication far exceeds his financial means. The medication remains in the pharmacy. He returns to the old couch and cigarette smoke. Two days later, with severe shortness of breath, he is taken by ambulance to the emergency department where he needs high-level care and a three-day hospital stay. Thus the patient's initial encounter, while quick, was by no means efficient when we factor in his subsequent course and need for tertiary healthcare.

HISTORY RECEIVING

Now contrast history taking with history receiving. History receiving roughly aligns with the patient-centered interview and is patient-driven. It acknowledges the patient as a partner in healthcare. The communication is open-ended and evolves, thereby allowing the health professional to appreciate the dynamic nature of illness within the patient's life (Fortin, Dwamena, Frankel, & Smith, 2012). Focus is on the patient rather than simply the disease. In the case of our young man with new onset non-productive cough and chest tightness, if the health professional invited his story with a statement such as, "Tell me about your living situation," and received the patient's history with curiosity, attention, and kindness, the patient may have had a different outcome. Certainly, there would have been opportunity for the health professional to hear about and intervene on the environmental triggers like dust and cigarette smoke. As importantly, "Tell me about your living situation" could have opened the door for the patient to talk about the violent relationship that drove him to live in an apartment with friends, and his now relentless feelings of fear, loss, and financial insecurity. Data supporting links among stress, emotional distress, grief, and physical illness are substantial (Cohen et al., 2012; Irwin, 2008). With the patient's story as a guide, the health professional may have recognized that in addition to environmental triggers for reactive airway disease, the patient had emotional precipitants for his illness that needed to be acknowledged and addressed, and financial concerns that warranted assistance to purchase his medications. The health professional receiving the history does not have to be the person who addresses the patient's psychosocial issues. That said, he or she must listen to the patient's story, acknowledge the psychosocial challenges, and engage appropriate staff to help the patient.

DETERMINANTS OF HEALTH

As health professionals, in order to hear and interpret patients' stories competently, we must understand the determinants of health. The determinants of health are a broad strokes approach to answering the question – why are some people healthy and others not? In the United States, the Healthy People initiatives, under the auspices of the Department of Health and Human Services in collaboration with health agencies and public stakeholders, provide health improvement objectives for the nation. These objectives are based on best available evidence and are updated every ten years. Healthy People 2020 identifies four categories of health determinants: biology and genetics, individual behavior, social and physical environment, and health services. I describe each category briefly here, and then focus on the social and physical environment, also called the social determinants of health (Healthy People 2020, 2018).

- **Biology and Genetics** is where the healthcare industry traditionally focuses money and attention. This category includes constitutional features such as anatomy, physiology, metabolism, age, sex, and inherited genetic factors.
- **Individual Behavior** includes dietary habits, physical activity, smoking, receiving recommended immunizations and screening tests, as well activities like using a condom, seatbelt, and bicycle helmet. In other words, the health promoting and protective activities that a person does or does not do.
- **Social and Physical Environment** encompasses a person's access to social and economic opportunities. These include the resources and supports available in someone's home, neighborhood, and community, the quality of the educational system, the safety of neighborhoods and workplaces, water, food, and air cleanliness, and the nature of social interactions and relationships.
- **Health Services** refers to access to healthcare and health insurance, adequacy of the healthcare workforce in terms of medical knowledge but also communication skills, healthcare quality assurance and patient safety, and cultural awareness.

Each of the four categories listed earlier influences and inter-relates with the other categories. This means optimal health outcomes depend upon patients and health professionals addressing all four categories – which may involve multiple health and social service professionals. In the context of this chapter, I focus on the social and physical environment category since this is a large generative pool for the patient's illness story. I encourage the reader to keep the other three categories, Biology and Genetics, Individual Behavior, Health Services, in mind as you read the Social and Physical Environment/Social Determinants of Health section.

SOCIAL AND PHYSICAL ENVIRONMENT/SOCIAL DETERMINANTS OF HEALTH

According to the World Health Organization (n.d.),

The social determinants of health are the conditions in which people are born, grow, live, work and age. These circumstances are shaped by the distribution of money, power and resources at global, national and local levels.

Social determinants of health are equivalent to the Healthy People 2020 category, Social and Physical Environment. Social factors, like family, culture and religion, neighbors, and the larger community, affect a person's health by encouraging or deterring social engagement and one's sense of security and safety. In addition, these factors determine one's susceptibility to the consequences of discrimination and racism. Factors from the physical environment similarly entwine with health. One's physical environment most directly correlates with economic status. The higher one's income, the more likely one is to live in a home free of environmental toxins, and in a neighborhood free of crime and violence. In the United States, neighborhood dictates access to public education, public transportation, variety and quality of food, and response times of public safety and emergency personnel. In addition, the physical environment affects quality of life by encouraging socialization and physical activity by the presence of streetlights, sidewalks, bike lanes, parks and ball fields, community centers, libraries, trash pick-up, and adaptations for people with disabilities (Center for Disease Control and Prevention, 2018).

THE NATIONAL HEALTH INTERVIEW SURVEY

In an effort to capture epidemiologic data about the health of the civilian population in the United States, the National Center for Health Statistics regularly conducts the National Health Interview Survey. The survey is administered annually to a sample consisting of approximately 40,000 households and 100,000 individuals. The survey provides a wealth of information connecting health and socioeconomic characteristics, and quantitatively substantiates the social determinants of health (National Center for Health Statistics, 2017a).

The survey asks questions like,

> During the past 12 months was there any time when you needed medical care but did not get it because you couldn't afford it?
>
> During the past 12 months has medical care been delayed because of worry about the cost?
>
> During the past 12 months was there any time when you needed prescription medicine but didn't get it because you couldn't afford it?

The National Health Interview Survey year on year trend data shows that lower educational attainment is a primary predictor of reduced healthcare access and prescription medication access (National Center for Health Statistics, 2017b). This means that the number of years someone spends in school directly aligns with that person's ability to gain access to healthcare services and medication.

MEDICATION ACCESS

Reduced prescription medication access is a leading cause of medication non-adherence, and is remarkably common in the United States. Research indicates approximately 25%–50% of patients do not fill their medication prescription or vary the dose and/or frequency of medication that they take from that which was instructed by their health professional (DiMatteo, 2004; Nieuwlaat et al., 2014). Among the primary reasons patients state for medication non-adherence are prohibitive costs of medication, fear of side effects, and belief that the medication will not be helpful (Boston Consulting Group, 2003; Kennedy, Tuleu, & Mackay, 2008) – reasons that have persisted for decades.

Let's think about implications of the medication non-adherence data. Patients seek help from a health professional, and yet when the health professional offers help in the form of a prescription medication, many of the patients will not follow through on the recommendation. And three of the primary reasons they will not follow through – financial barriers, fear, and disbelief that the medication will be helpful – could, in many cases, be readily addressed by open dialogue with the health professional. If we are receiving our patients' stories, we are positioned to hear about the economic circumstances that force them to choose between food, rent, and medicine – and we can engage the system to intervene on behalf of the patient. When we are open to our patients' stories, we are curious about their fears and beliefs, even when these do not appear on a checklist or dropdown menu.

EDUCATIONAL ATTAINMENT AND HEALTH

Data indicate that people with less than a high school diploma are several times more likely to be obese, smoke, be physically inactive, and have a higher incidence of diabetes and heart disease than more educated individuals (Center on Society and Health, 2018). The ultimate health outcome measure is, of course, mortality. Number of years of education predicts the odds of adult mortality. Furthermore, there are radical jumps in the mortality odds ratio across years of education. The most dramatic decrease in the odds of mortality occur at the critical juncture of obtaining a high school diploma, followed by a precipitous decrease in the odds of mortality with each additional year of education attained thereafter (Hummer & Hernandez, 2013). For the well-being of society, higher education cannot be a privilege afforded to some and not others, nor can it be catalogued as a social service independent of a nation's health. The evidence clearly demonstrates that education is a commanding determinant of health.

SOCIAL DETERMINANTS OF HEALTH: ADVOCACY AND CHANGE

Data implicate the deleterious health effects of low educational attainment and other social determinants such as decrepit housing, financial instability, inability to access quality food, and exposure to violence. The consequences of social determinants are an unambiguous and shameful statement about national priorities. Although illness may be a consequence of these social factors, it is also a magnifier. Physical and mental illness bring increased vulnerability, decreased capacity, and increased demands on resources, thus heightening the impact of social challenges. It is therefore all the more vital that we listen to our patients stories and understand the everyday struggles that comprise their lives. As health professionals, we can influence policy-makers and legislators to attend to social challenges and thereby improve our patients' health. By receiving the patient's history, we are not only better prepared to offer truly effective and efficient healthcare, we are also positioned to advocate for social changes that will improve health and well-being for all.

TYPES OF ILLNESS STORIES

Medical sociologist Arthur Frank, PhD (2013) contends that when the patient is the storyteller, the dominant sociocultural perception of illness shifts from passivity – where the ill person is a victim of disease and recipient of care (described in chapter 1, Illness Narratives section) – to one in which the patient is an active participant and partner in care. Professor Frank describes three types of illness stories: the restitution narrative, the chaos narrative, and the quest narrative, each of which I briefly describe here. The restitution narrative has a storyline that begins in a past state of health, describes the current illness including procedures and appointments, and concludes with a prediction for restored health. One example of the restitution narrative is the perky, cheerful, hopeful story that is prevalent on social media. The chaos narrative is an anxiety-riddled story of loss of control. The patient is overwhelmed and perceives the healthcare system and/or health professionals as unable to control the symptoms and disease, and perceives his/her own inability to control life's course. These are stories of vulnerability, frailty, desperation, and loneliness, with no obvious trajectory. In the quest narrative, the patient is a proactive arbiter who is on an illness journey. The patient self-identifies as chief executive officer of the healthcare team and sees the health professionals as employees, devoted to finding the optimal outcome. The patient claims agency to exert effort and control over his or her disease and is confident the illness journey itself has transformative value.

EFFECT OF STORY ON THE HEALTH PROFESSIONAL

What effect does receiving our patients' stories have on us as health professionals? Physician and anthropologist, Arthur Kleinman, MD (1988) posits that among the clinician's primary tasks are to receive our patient's story, and validate and affirm the value of the patient's experiences. These seemingly simple tasks are, at present, rare occurrences during the clinical encounter. There is an abundance of studies and commentary on patient-clinician communication; however, the vast majority of these publications either report patient satisfaction levels or quantify the health professional's communication deficiencies (Institute for Healthcare Communication, 2011). Researchers have documented the degradation in patient outcomes that occurs when health professionals circumnavigate the patient's story, including the consequent decline in patient trust, adherence, satisfaction, and safety. What is more difficult to find in the literature is the health professional's experience, both positive and negative, of hearing patients' stories.

In my experience, when I am able to connect with my patient, human to human, and engage with the illness story, the effect is profound and poignant. As a witness to my patients' stories I perform an essential role in helping my patients find meaning in their illness. In doing so, I also find meaning in my own work (see chapter 4 Bearing Witness to Suffering). With the art of history receiving, health professionals can be liberated from the technical role of data gathering and progress to the creative activities of healthcare, such as emotional engagement, self-expression, spontaneity, relationship building, and for some, spiritual practice. When we give ourselves the freedom to receive, attend to, synthesize, and interpret our patients' stories, we access our core human qualities and values.

In *Narrative Medicine: Honoring the Stories of Illness*, Rita Charon, MD, PhD (2006, p. 4) describes the multi-level, creative process of listening to a patient's story.

> I had to follow the patient's narrative thread, identify the metaphors or images used in the telling, tolerate ambiguity and uncertainty as the story unfolded, identify the unspoken subtexts, and hear one story in light of others told by this teller. . . . I also had to be aware of my own response to what I heard, allowing myself to be personally moved to action on behalf of the patient. I was the interpreter of these accounts of events of illness that are, by definition, unruly and elusive.

Receiving a patient's history, and everything associated with it, including, attention, openness, curiosity, and the complex cognitive processing necessary to synthesize the story, is nothing short of a creative act. Dr. Charon (2006, p. 188) goes on to say, "I find tremendous interest and joy in allowing myself to be bathed in a stranger's telling of self. I am stunned at how singular – how absolutely unique – are these self/body narratings."

Our patients' stories become a balm for our own lives, personal and professional, reminding us of our frailty and vulnerability, as well as our inherent capacity for empathy and compassion. This is our opportunity to use our empathic imagination to expand our vision beyond the aggressive, disease battle metaphor of the sociocultural illness narrative (see chapter 1 Introduction to Health Humanities, Illness Language and Narratives section), and instead to distill meaning from illness. We revisit these opportunities in more detail in chapter 6 Recognizing Our Interdependence.

THE PATIENT'S VOICE

In her 1926 essay, *On Being Ill*, Virginia Woolf (2002) ponders the absence of illness as a central component of story. Ms. Woolf contends that we have a paucity of language sufficient to convey the experience of illness. Nearly a century after Ms. Woolf's observations, there is a movement to amplify the patient's voice. Over the past couple of decades, concurrent with the ubiquity of the internet and social media, patient bloggers, advocacy groups, as well as healthcare systems and organizations have created space for patients to tell their stories. There are literally thousands of these sites on the internet with new ones appearing regularly. Of course, many are not peer-reviewed or endorsed by august institutions, leading one to question their quality and veracity, and raising concerns about the potential for patient harm. Some, however, have brilliantly merged the patient's voice with biomedical safeguards. The results are impressive. Here are a few examples.

The non-profit organization, Patients' View Institute (PVI) (2017), is committed to the "democratization of health care" as a means of improving healthcare quality. Their aim is to capture and disseminate patient narratives so that other patients, family members, health professionals, and biomedical industry leaders can learn from the stories. PVI also uses patient stories to advocate for policy and legislation to optimize safe, patient-centered healthcare delivery. Patient storytellers share their experiences with illness in the context of the rest of their lives, and are empowered to value and appreciate the effect their stories can have on finding solutions to systems-level healthcare problems.

DIPEx International (n.d.) is a partnership of academic institutions and non-profit organizations that combine efforts to conduct, analyze, and publish interviews with patients, families, and caregivers. Their website, healthtalk.org, features video and audio extracts from the interviews. DIPEx International aims to use rigorous qualitative methods and researcher mentorship, supervision, and training to assure quality and integrity are maintained while capturing people's stories of health and illness.

PatientsLikeMe (2018) is a repository for quantitative data provided by patients about their symptoms, treatment options, side effects, and "the real-world nature of disease." In addition, it is a network for patients to connect with others and share their narrative about living with illness. This unique dataset, generated by more than 500,000 patients, is advancing the biomedical industry and improving the care health professionals provide to patients.

Stanford physician Bassam Kadry, MD, had not recognized until a few years ago, when his mother became ill, the challenges patients and family members experience within the healthcare system. Since 2012, Dr. Kadry's family foundation has sponsored patients to join academicians, clinicians, technologists, and innovators at the Stanford University Medicine X conference. "Medicine X is a catalyst for new ideas about the future of medicine and health care. The initiative explores how emerging technologies will advance the practice of medicine, improve health, and empower patients to be active participants in their own care" (Stanford Medicine, n.d.). Dr. Kadry's goal is to prioritize patient perspective and experience in the drive to change healthcare (Stanford Medicine, 2013).

The 100,000 Lives Campaign, launched by the Institute for Healthcare Improvement (n.d.) to improve patient safety and increase healthcare efficiency, aims to apply evidence-based best practices at healthcare institutions across the United States to "extend or save as many as 100,000 lives" per year. The United Kingdom's National Health Service (n.d.) in Wales initiated The 1000 Lives Campaign, a comprehensive approach to patient safety and healthcare quality improvement modeled after The 100,000 Lives initiative. One part of The 1000 Lives Campaign acknowledges the value of the patient as storyteller. The National Health Service in Wales reports patient storytelling can be useful as inspiration for healthcare providers, as well as other patients. In addition, the patient perspective on environment, process, and communication within an institution can be helpful for systems-level improvements in healthcare.

Dave deBronkart, co-founder of the Society for Participatory Medicine and survivor of stage IV renal cancer, is a passionate and articulate advocate for patient engagement in healthcare. His goal is to modulate the subordinate role patients assume and the elevated role health professionals acquire in our paternalistic biomedical culture. Mr. deBronkart asserts that patients are an underused, valuable, and vital resource with much to add to the health professional's expertise. In his book, *Let Patients Help! A Patient Engagement Guide*, Mr. deBronkart (2013) describes ten ways patients can participate in improving healthcare. With the aim to whet your appetite for Mr. deBronkart's full-throated justification and appeal for these methods, I list his 10 patient participation recommendations here:

1   allow patients access to their medical data;
2   involve family caregivers, especially since they provide the bulk of the care between healthcare visits. Give family caregivers a way to enter information on the patient's chart;
3   encourage patients and families to search for medical information online. Help by alerting them to indicators of quality information;
4   urge patients and families to be attentive to potential errors and to speak up. For example, in the hospital, family members can provide health professionals with reminders about hand washing, and ask for confirmation on medications and dosages prior to delivery;
5   let patients know the cost of care, be it laboratory studies, diagnostic imaging, vaccinations, procedures, etc;
6   give patients a vote on the value of medical spending;
7   inform patients about who are the best providers by advertising success rates, complications, death rates, convenience, service, and patient satisfaction;
8   inform patients about the options that are available for any healthcare decision;
9   let patients help set the biomedical research agenda;
10 listen to how patients describe patient-centered care and adapt.

THE SUPPRESSED VOICE

The organizations previously described, and a growing number of others, are making impressive inroads in amplifying the patient's voice within healthcare. However, the patient's voice most often heard in the United States is white, educated, and English-speaking. We must remain cognizant of the suppressed voice. As health professionals, we interact with people from all walks of life on a daily basis. If we are attentive and open, we can hear stories from people that rarely receive a platform in our society, and elevate those stories for broader consideration. With an expansive understanding of patients' experiences with illness and the role of illness in people's complicated lives, we can become agents for social change.

CLOSING

In this chapter, we explored the impact of the patient storyteller on the patient, the health professional, and the healthcare industry. We looked at different types of illness stories that patients tell, and the essential need to be attentive to all the determinants of someone's health within the story, not simply the biological determinants. We considered the privilege afforded health professionals who understand patients' physical and social environments, and the opportunity for health professionals to be agents of social change. Finally, we looked at a few examples of forums where patients are using their illness stories to influence healthcare quality improvement.

With the elements of the chapter in mind, I provide learning objectives and activities for the reader to experience and reflect upon the idea of the patient as storyteller.

ACTIVITIES

LEARNING OBJECTIVES

Learners will

1 demonstrate the capacity of stories to affect an individual's behavior, interpretation of experiences, and distillation of meaning and purpose;
2 recognize how shared stories help construct relationships, societies, and cultural norms.

ESSAY AND DISCUSSION

First, read the essay, *Desperately Seeking Herb Weinman*, by Steven Lewis (2013). The essay is available at *https://pulsevoices.org/index.php/archive/stories/115-desperately-seeking-herb-weinman*. As you read, note words or passages that appeal to you, repel you, resonate with you, startle you, or in some way catch your attention. Drawing on material presented in chapter 2, reflect on the effect story has on the behaviors and experiences of people in the essay.

SMALL GROUP DISCUSSION

Learners are invited to discuss their experience with the essay. Whenever possible, learners should refer to specific passages in the essay. In particular, learners should aim to comment on the effect of story on Mr. Lewis's behavior and interpretation of experiences, as well as that of the health professionals. Faculty facilitators may choose to ask someone to read aloud a passage from the story that captured their attention. Reading aloud makes the text a presence in the room and helps everyone focus. If at all possible, allow the conversation about the text to evolve organically, directed by the learners' curiosity.

NOTE: **Appendix A** has general guidelines for facilitating a health humanities seminar. **Appendix B** has instruction and discussion prompts specific to this activity for faculty facilitators to use if learners are not able to initiate a robust discussion.

WRITING AND SHARING

The second activity is for the learner to write to a prompt that directly links the chapter content and the essay. Here is a suggested writing prompt:

> Recount a story from your youth that shaped your idea of what it means to be a health professional.

Faculty facilitators can invite the learners to share what they have written with the group. Learners should never be required to share their writings.

REFERENCE LIST

Boston Consulting Group. (2003). *The hidden epidemic: Finding a cure for unfilled prescriptions and missed doses.* Author. Retrieved from www.bcg.com/documents/file14265.pdf

Center for Disease Control and Prevention. (2018). *Social determinants of health: Know what affects health.* Author. Retrieved from www.cdc.gov/socialdeterminants/

Center on Society and Health. (2018). *Education and health initiative.* Virginia Commonwealth University. Retrieved from http://societyhealth.vcu.edu/work/the-projects/educationhealth.html

Charon, R. (2006). *Narrative medicine: Honoring the stories of illness.* New York: Oxford University Press.

Cohen, S., Janicki-Devert, D., Doyle, W. J., Miller, G. E., Frank, E., Rabin, B. S., & Turner, R. B. (2012). Chronic stress, glucocorticoid receptor resistance, inflammation, and disease risk. *Proceedings of the National Academy of Sciences of the USA, 109*(16), 5995–5999.

deBronkart, D. (2013). *Let patients help! A patient engagement guide.* Charleston, NC: CreateSpace Independent Publishing Platform.

DIPEx International. (n.d.). *About us.* Author. Retrieved from http://www.dipexinternational.org/about-us/

DiMatteo, M. R. (2004). Variations in patients' adherence to medical recommendations: A quantitative review of 50 years of research. *Medical Care, 42*(3), 200–209.

Fortin, A. H., Dwamena, F. C., Frankel, R. M., & Smith, R. C. (2012). *Smith's patient-centered interviewing: An evidence-based method* (3rd ed.). New York and Chicago, IL: McGraw-Hill.

Frank, A. (2013). *The wounded storyteller: Body, illness, and ethics* (2nd ed.). Chicago, IL: University of Chicago Press.

Gilbert, D. (2007). *Stumbling on happiness.* New York and Toronto: Random House.

Healthy People 2020. (2018). *Determinants of health.* Office of Disease Prevention and Health Promotion. Retrieved from www.healthypeople.gov/2020/about/foundation-health-measures/Determinants-of-Health

Hummer, R. A., & Hernandez, E. M. (2013). The effect of educational attainment on adult mortality in the United States. *Population Bulletin, 68*(1), 1–16.

Institute for Healthcare Communication. (2011). *Impact of communication in healthcare.* Author. Retrieved from http://healthcarecomm.org/about-us/impact-of-communication-in-healthcare/

Institute for Healthcare Improvement. (n.d.). *Overview of the 100,000 lives campaign.* Author. Retrieved from www.ihi.org/Engage/Initiatives/Completed/5MillionLivesCampaign/Documents/Overview%20of%20the%20100K%20Campaign.pdf

Irwin, M. R. (2008). Human psychoneuroimmunology: 20 years of discovery. *Brain, Behavior, and Immunity, 22,* 129–139.

Kennedy, J., Tuleu, I., & Mackay, K. (2008). Unfilled prescriptions of Medicare beneficiaries: Prevalence, reasons, and types of medicines prescribed. *Journal of Managed Care Pharmacy, 14*(6), 553–560.

Kleinman, A. (1988). *The illness narratives: Suffering, healing, and the human condition.* New York: Basic Books.

Lewis, S. (2013). Desperately seeking Herb Weinman. *Pulse: Voices from the Heart of Medicine.* Retrieved from https://pulsevoices.org/index.php/archive/stories/115-desperately-seeking-herb-weinman

National Center for Health Statistics. (2017a). *About the national health interview survey.* Center for Disease Control and Prevention. Retrieved from www.cdc.gov/nchs/nhis/about_nhis.htm

National Center for Health Statistics. (2017b). *National Health Interview Survey, 2016: Public-use data file and documentation.* Center for Disease Control and Prevention. Retrieved from www.cdc.gov/nchs/nhis/data-questionnaires-documentation.htm

National Health Service. (n.d.). *1000 lives improvement.* Author. Retrieved from www.1000livesplus.wales.nhs.uk/home

Nieuwlaat, R., Wilczynski, N., Navarro, T., Hobson, N., Jeffery, R., Keepanasseril, A., . . . Haynes, R. B. (2014). Interventions for enhancing medication adherence. *Cochrane Database of Systematic Reviews, 20*(11). doi:10.1002/14651858. CD000011.pub4

PatientsLikeMe. (2018). *About us.* Author. Retrieved from www.PatientsLikeMe.com/about

Patients' View Institute. (2017). *About PVI.* Author. Retrieved from https://gopvi.org/about/story

Stanford Medicine. (n.d.). *Medicine X: About.* Stanford University Press. Retrieved from https://medicinex.stanford.edu/about/

Stanford Medicine. (2013). *Medicine X: Bassam Kadry on the importance of amplifying the patient's voice at Medicine X.* Stanford University Press. Retrieved from https://medicinex.stanford.edu/2013/06/18/bassam-kadry-on-the-importance-of-amplifying-the-patient-voice-at-medicine-x/

Woolf, V. (2002). *On being ill.* Ashfield, MA: Paris Press.

World Health Organization. (n.d.). *Social determinants of health.* Author. Retrieved from www.who.int/social_determinants/sdh_definition/en/

3 UNCONSCIOUS BIAS

> INTEGRATION NOTE
> ....
> This chapter integrates with clinical skills training and cultural awareness
> curricula. The learner activity at the end of the chapter complements instruction
> related to nicotine addiction and smoking cessation.

INTRODUCTION

You have probably heard one or more of the following commonly held beliefs about
bias: People who exhibit bias toward or against someone are aware of their behavior; bias
and discrimination are behaviors practiced by immoral people; and those of us who are
upright people do not engage in discriminatory behavior. These three statements are not
true. Advances in neuroscience and social science demonstrate that *everyone* has biases.
Having biases is part of being human. We are naturally inclined to make microsecond
decisions about other people based on very little, superficial information. It is how we
make decisions about whether we are safe. Unfortunately, most of the time we are not
even aware of our biases. With startling frequency, we are unconscious of our biases and
the consequent discriminatory behavior we exhibit against one person and in favor of
someone else. Our unconscious biases can lead to considerable problems as we unwittingly
and unconsciously cause harm – especially to those who are depending on and expecting
our objectivity – namely, our patients.

In this chapter, I summarize the literature on unconscious bias, and then talk about
unconscious bias in the clinical setting. I share data on troubling patient outcomes that
occur when health professionals and healthcare systems have unchecked bias toward
certain populations. I describe conscious and deliberate steps we can take to increase
awareness of our biases and overcome them to provide optimal patient care. The chapter
concludes with activities that provide opportunity for experiential learning related to
unconscious bias.

THE SCIENCE OF UNCONSCIOUS BIAS

Our unconscious minds hold beliefs and attitudes that we would never consciously
endorse (Staats, 2014). For more than three decades, social scientists have been studying
unconscious bias, which refers to the beliefs and attitudes that activate involuntarily

without conscious awareness, and influence our thoughts and actions (Blair, 2002; Kang, 2012; Rudman, 2004). I want to emphasize that unconscious bias is not simply beliefs and attitudes that one suppresses or conceals because of fear of social reprisal. To suppress or conceal one's beliefs and attitudes requires conscious awareness and control. Unconscious bias is involuntary and beyond conscious awareness and control. In the literature, you will see the label implicit bias used interchangeably with unconscious bias. I prefer the term unconscious bias because it unambiguously highlights the unconscious origin of our beliefs and attitudes.

HOW DO OUR UNCONSCIOUS BIASES FORM?

Research indicates our unconscious biases derive from repeated messages we consume from news and entertainment media and our sociocultural group that associate particular characteristics with particular subpopulations (Kang, 2012). University of Massachusetts professor and social psychologist, Nilanjana Dasgupta, PhD (2013, p. 237) writes,

> commonly held opinions of social groups are known by everybody immersed in a given community through hearsay, media exposure, and by passive observation of who occupies valued roles and devalued roles in the community. Passive exposure to commonly held attitudes and beliefs register in individuals' minds and get incorporated into their mental representation of a given group without their active consent. As a result, people's implicit attitudes toward social groups often mirror the societal hierarchy of privilege and disadvantage.

With iterative exposures, we unconsciously pair characteristics with a subpopulation, independent of the veracity of the association. For example, largely due to the media and the passive observation that men hold the vast majority of positions of power and influence, about three out of every four United States citizens unconsciously link men with leadership and women with nurturance (Staats, Capatosto, Wright, & Jackson, 2016).

We can have biases for or against any number of characteristics including weight, sexual orientation, gender, religious affiliation, political party affiliation, sports team fan, employment status, nation of origin, race, ethnicity, literacy, primary language, verbal syntax, dialect, and accent – the list goes on and on. If we can sense a characteristic, we can form beliefs, attitudes, and biases toward and against that characteristic.

ASSESSMENT OF UNCONSCIOUS BIAS

Assessment of unconscious bias is a challenge since researchers are trying to extract information that participants do not even know they possess. Early studies assessed participants' physiologic response to stimuli. For example, several studies used functional magnetic resonance imaging (fMRI) to examine amygdala activation when participants were shown photographs of black people's faces and white people's faces (Cunningham et al., 2004; Lieberman, Hariri, Jarcho, Eisenberger, & Bookheimer, 2005; Phelps et al.,

2000). The amygdala is part of the brain's limbic system and is known to react to fear and other stimuli related to threat and danger. Another study used facial electromyography on participants while they viewed images of black and white people's faces to assess movement of the muscles activated when smiling and frowning (Vanman, Saltz, Nathan, & Warren, 2004).

At present, the most widely used assessment tool for unconscious bias is the Implicit Association Test (IAT). The IAT is a latency response measure that relies on reaction times to determine conceptual and evaluative associations (Greenwald, McGhee, & Schwartz, 1998). The IAT has been widely studied – when I entered the term "implicit association test" into the search engine, PubMed, I received more than 1,000 hits. From 1998 to 2015, over 12 million people took the internet-based, self-assessment IAT (C. Vitiello, personal communication, October 13, 2017). Within the research community, the IAT receives criticism primarily from those who question whether it is actually testing familiarity and cultural knowledge rather than unconscious bias (Arkes & Tetlock, 2004; Blanton, Strauts, Jaccard, Mitchell, & Tetlock, 2015; Ottaway, Hayden, & Oakes, 2001). Of note, the instrument performs well in psychometric testing, including reliability and estimates of validity (Kang & Lane, 2010). The IAT is particularly effective, and superior to self-report, at identifying bias around socially sensitive issues related to race, gender, ethnicity, sexual orientation, and age (Greenwald, Poehlman, Uhlmann, & Banaji, 2009). I encourage you to check out the IAT self-assessment tests available at *https://implicit. harvard.edu/implicit/takeatest.html* and learn more about Project Implicit, a multi-national, research network devoted to understanding unconscious bias and related constructs.

ACTIVATION OF UNCONSCIOUS BIAS

Our unconscious biases are more likely to activate if we are in a high intensity situation with competing cognitive demands and/or have to deal with time constraints (Reskin, 2005; Smedley, Stith, & Nelson, 2003). These three descriptors – high intensity situation, competing cognitive demands, and time constraints – also aptly describe clinical care. As health professionals, we must cope with a complicated healthcare system and workplace environment built for speed – which may inadvertently trigger our unconscious biases. In addition, as individuals, we must contend with our own exposures to messaging that shape our unconscious biases. Later in this chapter, I present ways we can intervene to mitigate our unconscious biases (see the section, How to Overcome Unconscious Bias).

UNCONSCIOUS BIAS IN THE CLINICAL SETTING

Now let's talk about the harm that comes to patients from bias in healthcare. The Institute of Medicine report entitled, *Unequal Treatment: Confronting Racial and Ethnic Disparities in Healthcare*, addressed the topic of health professional bias head on (Smedley et al.,

2003). The authors state "even at equivalent levels of access to care, racial and ethnic minorities experience a lower quality of health services and are less likely to receive even routine medical procedures than white Americans" (p. 29). The authors go on to say,

> Three mechanisms might be operative in producing discriminatory patterns of healthcare from the provider's side of the exchange: 1) bias (or prejudice) against minorities; 2) greater clinical uncertainty when interacting with minority patients; and 3) beliefs (or stereotypes) held by the provider about the behavior or health of minorities.
>
> (p. 161)

As you can imagine, this report caused quite a stir. It made healthcare professionals, including administrators, policy-makers, practitioners, and educators, take a hard and uncomfortable look at who we are, what we are doing, and how we can improve healthcare delivery in the United States. Unfortunately, we have made little progress since the report was published in 2003. Discrepancies in diagnosis and treatment for minority patients persist. The 2016 National Healthcare Quality and Disparities report shows black patients received worse care than white patients on 42% of quality measures, and Hispanic patients received worse care than white patients on 37% of quality measures. Trend data from 2000–2015 show the percentage of quality measures with disparities by race and ethnicity are largely unchanged over this time period (Agency for Healthcare Research and Quality, 2017).

Do the gross disparities on healthcare quality measures by race and ethnicity presented in the 2016 National Healthcare Quality and Disparities Report definitively point to health professional bias? The problem is, of course, much more complex than the single variable of health professional bias. That said, the data prompts us to pause, reflect, and consider our personal contribution to the discrepancies. In the following section, I present studies that link health professional unconscious bias to patient outcomes.

HEALTH PROFESSIONAL UNCONSCIOUS BIAS

During the past 15 years, research on unconscious bias among healthcare workers has escalated. I summarize here some representative studies. This is by no means a comprehensive literature review of unconscious bias in healthcare, but rather a sampling to provide the reader with an appreciation for the pervasiveness of unconscious bias and its consequences. To date, the preponderance of research on unconscious bias in healthcare uses physician participants.

RACE

Let's begin by looking at a study that compared physician unconscious bias to that of the general population. In 2009, Sabin, Nosek, Greenwald, and Rivara studied more than

400,000 participants to measure implicit and explicit attitudes about race using data from the internet-based, self-administered Implicit Association Test (IAT). Within this large study population was a sub-sample of 2,535 physicians. The physician subpopulation was no different from the entire study population in showing an unconscious preference for white Americans as compared to black Americans. Physicians and the general study population were also similar in having their unconscious bias exceed their explicit endorsement of white preference. When the researchers looked at the results by physician race and ethnicity, they found white physicians showed the strongest implicit preference for white Americans. African-American physicians were unique among their physician peers in that they did not demonstrate an unconscious preference for either black or white Americans. Study results dichotomized by gender showed women physicians, of all races/ethnicities, demonstrated significantly less unconscious bias than men physicians did.

Of course, our concern is not with how physicians and other health professionals perform on a latency response test like the IAT, but rather with how unconscious biases leak into the realm of patient care. The diagnostic and treatment inequities endured by minorities are indisputable, as is the fact that all humans have some degree of unconscious biases. The question remains as to the contribution of health professionals' unconscious biases to healthcare inequities.

Shavers, Bakos, and Sheppard (2010) conducted a systematic review of the published literature to determine racial/ethnic patterns of pain management, attitudes toward pain, pain assessment, healthcare provider prescribing patterns, and community access to pain medications and other coping strategies. Using data from 187 studies, the authors report,

> Racial/ethnic minority patients are less likely than White patients to receive any pain medication, more likely to receive lower doses of pain medications, more likely to have longer wait times to receipt of pain medication in the emergency department, and less likely to receive opiates as treatment for pain despite higher pain scores, and to be treated in a manner consistent with the World Health Organization recommendations.
>
> (p. 179)

The authors found evidence for multiple determinants of discrepant pain management across racial/ethnic patient groups. For example, each culture group has distinct ways of expressing pain, both verbally and non-verbally. When the health professional and patient do not share a cultural understanding, the health professional may fail to believe and/or interpret properly the patient's pain expression. Analysis revealed disparate prescribing practices for racial/ethnic minority patients. Of note, the attitudes and beliefs of both health professionals and patients gave rise to the prescribing practices. Health professionals were overall reluctant to prescribe narcotic pain medication to minority patients for fear the patients would abuse the medications or become addicted. Interestingly, racial and ethnic minority patients were less inclined than their white counterparts were to accept narcotic pain medication because the minority patients feared becoming addicted.

Shavers et al. (2010) systematic review confirms detriment to patients caused by cultural ignorance and prompts the question: Is health professional cultural ignorance a precursor to unconscious bias or a form of unconscious bias? Health professionals and patients cannot wait for a scholarly answer to the question. Patient harm from healthcare disparities happens daily. As health professionals, we must each work to increase our awareness of our personal cultural ignorance and mollify the negative impact on patients.

A landmark study by Green et al. (2007) used the IAT to look at whether unconscious racial biases influenced physician referral of patients with acute coronary symptoms for thrombolysis. Results showed that although physicians did not explicitly endorse pro-white preferences, measurement of unconscious bias demonstrated preference for white patients. Physicians with the highest pro-white biases had the greatest likelihood of treating white patients, but not black patients, with thrombolysis. A similarly designed study of pediatricians found a direct correlation between the strength of unconscious pro-white preferences and the tendency to prescribe narcotics to white children in pain but not to prescribe narcotics for black children in pain (Sabin & Greenwald, 2012).

Haider et al. (2015) looked at the relationship between unconscious bias (race and social class) and clinical decisions made by 245 registered nurses who worked in the intensive care units, emergency department, and acute surgical units at Johns Hopkins Medical Center. Using the IAT, the researchers determined the nurses had significant unconscious pro-white and pro-upper social class preference, despite explicit endorsement of egalitarian views. The nurses viewed clinical vignettes of patients with post-operative pain, drug misuse, rib fracture, alcohol withdrawal, domestic violence, patient restraint, family relations, and eliciting patient consent. The patients depicted in the vignettes varied randomly by race and social class, with each nurse viewing two black and two white patients and two upper social class and two lower social class patients. After each clinical vignette, the nurses answered questions about how they would manage the patient. Results showed no relationship between the nurses' considerable unconscious bias and their clinical assessment and decision-making for vignette patients. Haider et al. note that results from this single study of nurses stand in contrast to several studies of physicians that directly link unconscious bias to altered patient care. The authors conclude,

> Results of the current study suggest that an additional mitigating factor might be involved in the relationship between a nurse's implicit preference toward white and higher social class patients and the manner in which he/she delivers care to his/her patients. For example, it is possible that some aspects of the RNs' training and/or their hands-on, on-the-job experience with a diverse group of patients might uniquely buffer nurses from the impact of implicit biases in a manner that differs from other providers.
>
> (p. 1084)

Certainly, we need additional rigorous studies of unconscious bias among nurses and other health professionals treating actual patients rather than vignettes before we can make definitive statements about equitable clinical decision making. However, while we await the accumulation of evidence, health inequities persist in the United States. It behooves us to investigate nursing education to see what elements contribute to equitable clinical decision making that can, in turn, translate to educational programs for other health professionals.

In 2017, researchers conducted a systematic review of nine studies that used the IAT and assessed physician clinical decision making (Dehon et al., 2017). Similar to the prior literature, all nine studies showed an unconscious pro-white preference. The relationship between unconscious bias and clinical decision making, however, was minimal among the studies – only two of the nine studies demonstrated an association between unconscious bias and discriminatory clinical decisions. Of note, eight of the nine studies used clinical vignettes rather than actual patient outcomes. It is possible unconscious bias does not affect clinical decision making with a vignette in the same way that it might affect actual patient care because real-time triggers, such as high intensity situations, competing cognitive demands, and time pressure, are not in play.

At present, we know relatively little about the influence of unconscious bias on patient care. There is a paucity of research about the unconscious biases of health professionals other than physicians. I encourage the interested reader to consider contributing to this burgeoning research. The potential to learn across professions is high.

WHO IS VULNERABLE TO HEALTH PROFESSIONALS' BIAS?

Lest you think unconscious bias in healthcare is exclusively about race and ethnicity, there is a growing literature about health professionals' biases against patients who are obese, transgender, women, and those who have mental illness (James et al., 2016; Phelan et al., 2015; Society for Women's Health Research, 2017; Thornicroft, Rose, & Kassam, 2007). Independent of the literature, each of us will bring our own unique biases to clinical care. Maybe our biases are against people who smoke, or people who are extreme athletes, or people with multiple sexual partners, or people with economic privilege – the possibilities for our personal biases are endless. It is incumbent upon us to be aware of our biases so we can mitigate negative effects for our patients.

Following is a sampling of epidemiologic studies, controlled trials, and qualitative studies that report untoward outcomes among three patient populations vulnerable to health professionals' bias: women, transgender people, and individuals who have mental illness.

WOMEN

Several studies demonstrate the under-diagnosis of coronary heart disease in women. Each time study results showed physicians were failing to diagnosis women with coronary heart disease, reviewers and readers offered explanations, such as women did not present with distinct symptoms or women declined diagnostic studies that would help make the diagnosis. No one proposed the possibility that physicians might have gender bias. Then scientists designed a controlled study (Maserejian, Link, Lutfey, Marceau, & McKinlay, 2009) in which physicians watched video vignettes of men and women presenting with identical symptoms and asked physicians to give their most certain diagnosis. Physicians were significantly less certain of a coronary heart disease diagnosis for women than for men, and 31.3% of the time the physicians said their most certain diagnosis for women was a mental health condition. Again, women in the study presented with the exact same symptoms as their male counterparts; patient gender was the only difference in the vignettes. Yet, instead of recognizing women's symptoms as most likely relating to a coronary heart disease diagnosis, nearly a third of the time, physicians were most certain women were mentally ill. The results of this study indicate physicians are not immune to the insidious negative messages our news, entertainment media, and cultural sources feed us about women (Jamieson, 2014). The potency of the negative messaging is such that it can override rigorous medical training and commitment to professionalism.

Now let's look at a recent study that used actual patients to determine treatment patterns by gender for cardiovascular disease. When a patient presents with ST-segment elevation myocardial infarction the standard of care is to treat with balloon angioplasty with the goal of revascularization. The shorter the length of time from patient presentation to insertion of the balloon (referred to as "door-to-balloon time"), the less patient morbidity and mortality. A 2013 Australian study of 735 patients presenting with ST-segment elevation myocardial infarction found, even after adjusting for covariates, women had a 13% increase in median door-to-balloon time compared to men (Dreyer et al., 2013). Other studies have found that women are less likely than men are to receive interventions to prevent and treat cardiovascular disease. Gender disparities extend to cholesterol screening and treatment, use of blood thinners during myocardial infarction, antiplatelet therapy for secondary prevention of cardiovascular disease, and implantation of cardioverter-defibrillators (Society for Women's Health Research, 2017).

A recent prospective study from The Netherlands examined how effective nurses were at assessing pain for patients who presented to the emergency department with musculoskeletal injury (Pierik, IJzerman, Gaakeer, Vollenbroek-Hutten, & Doggen, 2017). Of the 539 adult patients in the study, nurses were concordant with patient self-assessment of pain a mere 27% of the time. Within the discordant data, nurses judged the patient's pain to be significantly less than patient self-report 63% of the time. Nurses were much more likely to underestimate pain experienced by women than that experienced by men.

The 2017 Center for Medicare and Medicaid Services report, *Racial and Ethnic Disparities by Gender in Healthcare in Medicare Advantage*, shows women are significantly less likely than men are to receive referral for alcohol or other drug treatment. These results stand across the racial and ethnic groups described (white, black, Asian/Pacific Islander, and Hispanic). Similar to the evidence about cardiovascular disease management and pain assessment, disparate referral for alcohol and drug treatment based on gender is incongruous with our professional claim of egalitarian care, and yet the disparity is real and substantial.

For a detailed discussion of gender health and healthcare disparities, I direct the reader to the Society for Women's Health Research website (http://swhr.org/). The Society for

Women's Health Research is a non-profit organization that promotes research on biological differences in disease with the goal of "advancing women's health through science, advocacy, and education." For a sophisticated and nuanced exploration of cultural depictions and distortions of women's pain, I refer the reader to the essay, *Grand Unified Theory of Female Pain* by Leslie Jamieson (2014) and *The Cancer Journals* by Audre Lorde (1997).

TRANSGENDER PEOPLE

Transgender people are a comparatively understudied population. Until recently, most of the research has focused almost exclusively on HIV/AIDS and other sexually transmitted infections, while neglecting the general health needs of transgender people (Harvey & Housel, 2014). This void in the research literature is a form of institutional bias that the Institute of Medicine (2011) and Healthy People 2020 (2018) aim to rectify. The Institute of Medicine and Healthy People 2020 have each issued a call for increased research. Healthy People 2020 delineated a series of objectives to increase population-based data systems which collect data on (or for) lesbian, gay, bisexual, and transgender populations and correlate that data with health outcomes and health behaviors.

Despite the current dearth of research, we still find evidence of health disparities for transgender people. The first large scale national survey of transgender people occurred in 2008 when the National Center for Transgender Equality and the National Gay and Lesbian Task Force joined expertise to create and launch the National Transgender Discrimination Survey of 7,000 transgender people (Grant et al., 2010). Results showed transgender people are at high risk to misuse drugs or alcohol

> specifically to cope with the discrimination they faced due to their gender identity or expression. . . . A staggering 41% of respondents reported attempting suicide compared to 1.6% of the general population, with unemployment, low income, and sexual and physical assault raising the risk factors significantly.
>
> (p. 1)

In addition, the survey findings shed a harsh light on the healthcare industry. Nearly one in five respondents report being denied care because they are transgender or gender non-conforming. American Indians report the highest refusal of care because they are transgender or gender non-conforming at 36% of respondents. Of note, 28% of respondents report being the victim of harassment in medical settings, and 50% report having to educate their healthcare provider about transgender care. I ask the reader to pause and process these statistics. The transgender people who responded to this survey sought help from health professionals. Instead of help, a large percentage of transgender patients experienced harassment and ignorance.

The 2015 United States Transgender Survey is the largest survey of transgender adults to date with 27,715 respondents from all 50 states, the District of Columbia, American Samoa, Guam, Puerto Rico, and US military bases overseas (James et al., 2016). Summer 2015, the National Center for Transgender Equality conducted the study as an anonymous, online survey available in English and Spanish. The published report of the 2015 United States Transgender Survey provides a detailed look at experiences of transgender people with education, employment, family life, health, housing, and interactions with the criminal justice system. In the seven years since the National Transgender Discrimination Survey (described earlier) there has been little or no evidence of improvement in health and healthcare for transgender people. Results show transgender people endure serious psychological distress (39%) at a much higher rate compared to the overall United States population (5%). "Among the starkest findings is that 40% of respondents have attempted suicide in their lifetime – nearly nine times the attempted suicide rate in the U.S. population (4.6%)" (p. 9). Discriminatory practices by health professionals toward transgender people persist at a disturbing rate. We can do better. Understanding our biases and ignorance is a first step toward being able to provide decent, quality healthcare.

For the reader interested in addressing transgender bias in healthcare at the systems level, I encourage you to explore the Human Rights Campaign (n.d.) *Healthcare Equality Index*. Here you will find instruments and national benchmarks that you can apply at your healthcare institution.

PEOPLE WHO HAVE MENTAL ILLNESS

The American Psychiatric Association (2018) defines mental illness as

> health conditions involving changes in thinking, emotion or behavior (or a combination of these). Mental illnesses are associated with distress and/or problems functioning in social, work or family activities.

The most common diagnoses included under the heading of mental illness are major depressive disorder, schizophrenia, bipolar disorder, panic disorder, post-traumatic stress disorder, and obsessive-compulsive disorder.

PREVALENCE

Let's take a moment to understand the pervasive presence of mental illness within society. The World Health Organization periodically collects data about mental illness by conducting face-to-face surveys of approximately 60,000 households across 28 countries in the Americas, Europe, Middle East, Africa, and Asia (Kessler et al., 2009). The surveys show wide variation in mental illness prevalence by country; it is unclear if this is a function of variable disclosure practices secondary to culture and stigma, or true prevalence. That said, mental illness imposes a considerable global burden of disease (World Health Organization, 2011).

All subpopulations are susceptible to mental illness regardless of race/ethnicity or socioeconomic status. However, the World Health Organization Mental Health Action Plan identifies the following subpopulations as being at increased risk for developing mental illness: individuals who are impoverished, living with chronic health conditions, living in isolation, exposed to serious adversity as a child, experiencing human rights violations, and those exposed to war (World Health Organization, 2013).

One of many stark and sobering findings from the World Mental Health Surveys is the paucity of care available to people with serious mental illness. In developed countries, 35.5% to 50.3% of people with serious mental illness received no treatment in the previous 12-month period. These numbers swell to 76.3% to 85.4% of people with serious mental illness in less-developed countries (Kessler et al., 2009).

HOW DO HEALTH PROFESSIONALS CONTRIBUTE TO BIAS AGAINST PEOPLE WITH MENTAL ILLNESS?

Graham Thornicroft, Professor of Community Psychiatry, King's College London, has made significant contributions to our understanding of health professional discriminatory practices against people with mental illness (Thornicroft, 2006; Thornicroft et al., 2007). Professor Thornicroft describes two important factors that drive the negative attitudes patients with mental illness encounter in healthcare: physician bias (which I believe applies to other health professions as well), and diagnostic overshadowing.

PHYSICIAN BIAS

Physician bias, as well as that of other health professionals, is rooted in clinical experience. The preponderance of our clinical exposure to people with mental illness is with those who are acutely ill, do not respond to treatment, do not fully recover, or relapse. We have little experience with people who respond to treatment and make a full recovery – because people who recover no longer present for mental illness care. Consequently, health professionals tend to have a negatively skewed and pessimistic view of mental illness prognosis that we unconsciously convey to patients (Thornicroft, 2006). A study conducted in Sweden explored and compared attitudes toward mental illness by mental health workers and their patients (Hansson, Jormfeldt, Svedberg, & Svensson, 2011). Researchers used the 12-item Perceived Devaluation-Discrimination Questionnaire to discern attitudes from mental health workers (primarily nurses) and patients. Results showed,

> In general, negative attitudes towards people with a mental illness were predominant among staff, with a majority having a negative attitude in six out of the 12 items and more than one-third in all 12 items. The most negative attitudes concerned whether an employer would pass over an application for work in favour of another applicant without mental illness (75.6%), whether most young women would be reluctant to date a man who had been hospitalized for a mental illness (67.4%) or would hire a former mental patient to take care of their children (66.4%). Patients of these services in most instances shared these negative attitudes and beliefs with the staff. . . . There was no significant difference between staff and patients in the sum score of the scale.

(p. 51)

In an effort to understand how patients experience mental illness discrimination, researchers in the United Kingdom conducted structured telephone interviews with people who use mental health services (Hamilton et al., 2014). Qualitative content analysis of the transcribed interviews revealed seven discriminatory practices: organizational decisions, mistreatment, social distancing, stereotyping, lack of understanding, dismissiveness, and overprotectiveness. The study underscores the challenges patients with mental illness experience from discriminatory practices.

DIAGNOSTIC OVERSHADOWING

Diagnostic overshadowing means the mental illness diagnosis eclipses the health professional's ability to identify other potential diagnoses – or as Abraham Maslow (1966, p. 15) writes, "I suppose it is tempting, if the only tool you have is a hammer, to treat everything as if it were a nail." Diagnostic overshadowing can lead to dire oversights and health consequences when we incorrectly presume the patient's signs and symptoms relate to their mental illness and neglect to conduct a work up for a physical illness diagnosis (Thornicroft, 2006). Epidemiologic data repeatedly demonstrate excess morbidity and mortality for people with mental illness as compared to the general population (Kisely, Sadek, MacKenzie, Lawrence, & Campbell, 2008; Laursen, Munk-Olsen, & Gasse, 2011; Laursen, Nordentoft, & Mortensen, 2014). People with mental illness have up to seven times higher mortality rate as compared to the general population (Laursen, Munk-Olsen, Nordentoft, & Mortensen, 2007). Unfortunately, research has not yet exposed the degree to which diagnostic overshadowing contributes to the increased burden of disease and premature death experienced by people with mental illness. As I said earlier in this chapter, while we wait for evidence to accrue, we can commit to do better by our patients.

With the aim of discovering healthcare workers' perceptions of challenges involved in diagnosing people with mental illness, researchers conducted qualitative interviews with emergency department physicians and nurses at four hospitals in the United Kingdom (Shefer, Henderson, Howard, Murray, & Thornicroft, 2014). Thematic analysis of the transcribed interviews revealed multiple factors, as perceived by the physicians and nurses, lead to misdiagnosis or delayed treatment. Factors related directly to the patient include complex clinical presentations, frequent presentation to the emergency department, poor communication, and patient refusal of physical examination and/or diagnostic studies. Background factors include the emergency department environment (crowding and time pressures), as well as healthcare workers having negative attitudes toward people with mental illness. The authors conclude healthcare workers' discriminatory practices are only one of several factors that contribute to diagnostic overshadowing. That said, disparate treatment of people with mental illness is demoralizing, disrespectful, and preventable. With attention and effort, we can expunge discriminatory behavior from our professional relationships and optimize care for our patients.

HOW TO OVERCOME UNCONSCIOUS BIASES

Since the Institute of Medicine report, *Unequal Treatment: Confronting Racial and Ethnic Disparities in Healthcare*, there have been major initiatives to help health professionals and health professional students learn to bring their unconscious biases to consciousness. The research to date consistently shows that our unconscious biases are malleable. Through a process called de-biasing, embedded negative associations are replaced gradually with untarnished links (Dasgupta, 2013). De-biasing is neither easy nor quick, though with focused attention, awareness, and repeated effort, it is possible.

The first step to overcome our biases is to admit that we have them. Remember, we do not have biases because we are immoral, but rather because we are human. In order to admit we have biases, we have to first look for them and reflect on them – then we can work on overcoming them (see chapter 6 Recognizing our Interdependence, Mindfulness and Interbeing sections). Here are some de-biasing techniques that have robust research evidence to support their use (Staats, 2014; Staats et al., 2016).

Counter-stereotypic training: We can build new mental associations by providing visual and/or verbal cues that promote positive characteristics of the subpopulation that is perceived negatively. For example, to counter the barrage of media images that depict Arabs as boorish and violent, we can expose ourselves to visual cues of Arab men and women engaged in loving, caring, supportive, peaceful relationships.

Intergroup contact: As we saw by several of the research studies described in this chapter, ignorance plays a role in our biases. Interaction with members of the population that we perceive negatively can reduce our biases, as long as the interaction involves "individuals sharing equal status and common goals, a cooperative rather than competitive environment, and the presence of support from authority figures, laws, or customs" (Staats, 2014, p. 20).

Sense of accountability: If there are quality assurance structures in place that hold us accountable for our beliefs and behaviors toward our patients, then we are more likely to pause and limit the influence of habitual unconscious bias.

Deliberative processing: Unconscious biases can be offset by continuous self-monitoring of our habitual thinking, recognition of multiple viewpoints, and focusing on the unique traits of individuals rather than the demographic category to which they belong.

Meditation training: Effectiveness research on meditation training as an intervention for unconscious bias is still in its infancy. Early studies of loving-kindness meditation and mindfulness meditation favorably decreased unconscious bias in short-term follow-up (Kang, Grey, & Dovidio, 2014; Lueke & Gibson, 2015; Stell & Farsides, 2016). Since many forms of meditation, including loving-kindness and mindfulness, encompass non-judgmental awareness of the mind, it seems logical that meditation training will help mitigate habitual responses like unconscious bias. I look forward to more research in this area, especially with health professionals. For a fuller description of loving-kindness meditation see the section entitled Loving-kindness Meditation in chapter 4. For a fuller description of mindfulness see the section entitled Mindfulness in chapter 6.

CLOSING

In this chapter, we looked at the science of unconscious bias and its origin in the repeated messages we receive from news and entertainment media and our sociocultural group. We reviewed research that revealed health professionals are susceptible to potent social messaging such that it can override our professional education and commitment to egalitarian care. We saw the healthcare system and workplace environment as situationally primed to inadvertently trigger our unconscious biases. We learned from the data that cultural ignorance seems to have a role in fueling our biases, and confirmed the detriment to patients caused by our cultural ignorance. We looked at a sampling of the unconscious bias research and the untoward clinical outcomes experienced by racial/ethnic minorities, women, transgender people, and people with mental illness. Finally, we described conscious and deliberate steps we can take to increase awareness of our biases and overcome them to provide decent, equitable, respectful patient care.

I close this chapter with learning objectives and activities that provide the reader with the personal experience of unconscious bias. The activities allow you to observe your own biases without the competing demands of providing care to a patient, thus making your experience a personal learning laboratory on unconscious bias.

ACTIVITIES

LEARNING OBJECTIVES

Learners will

1 discuss the influence of unconscious bias in healthcare;
2 reflect on their personal biases.

VIDEO CLIP AND DISCUSSION

First, the learner watches the video clip, *Rebecca Berkowitz: My Quit Smoking Story* (Berkowitz, 2009), which is available at http://youtu.be/lNzirNkLods. As you watch, record words or behaviors that make you believe that Ms. Berkowitz will or will not quit smoking.

SMALL GROUP DISCUSSION
Learners are invited to discuss their experience with the video clip. Whenever possible, learners should refer to specific passages in the video clip that exemplify or trigger their discussion points. In particular, learners should aim to comment on how Ms. Berkowitz's appearance, expressed attitudes, and behaviors affect their belief that she will or will not

quit smoking. Learners should also consider any personal biases they have about Ms. Berkowitz's appearance, expressed attitudes, and behaviors that contribute to their belief about her ability or inability to quit smoking.

NOTE: **Appendix A** has general guidelines for facilitating a health humanities seminar. **Appendix B** has instruction and discussion prompts specific to this activity for faculty facilitators to use if your learners are not able to initiate a robust discussion.

WRITING AND SHARING

The second activity is for the learner to write to a prompt that directly links the chapter content and the short story. Here is a suggested writing prompt:

Describe a time when someone had a bias against you. Feel free to write fiction.

Faculty facilitators can invite the learners to share what they have written with the group. Learners should never be required to share their writings.

REFERENCE LIST

Agency for Healthcare Research and Quality. (2017). *2016 National healthcare quality and disparities report*. AHRQ Pub. No. 17–0001. Rockville, MD: Author. Retrieved from www.ahrq.gov/research/findings/nhqrdr/nhqdr16/index.html

American Psychiatric Association. (2018). *What is mental illness?* Author. Retrieved from www.psychiatry.org/patients-families/what-is-mental-illness

Arkes, H. R., & Tetlock, P. E. (2004). Attributions of implicit prejudice or would Jesse Jackson 'fail' the Implicit Association Test? *Psychological Inquiry, 15*, 257–278.

Berkowitz, E. (Producer). (2009). *Rebecca Berkowitz: My quit smoking story*. Retrieved from http://youtu.be/INzirNkLods

Blair, I. V. (2002). The malleability of automatic stereotypes and prejudice. *Personality and Social Psychology Review, 6*(3), 242–261.

Blanton, H., Strauts, E., Jaccard, J., Mitchell, G., & Tetlock, P. E. (2015). Towards a meaningful metric of implicit bias. *Journal of Applied Psychology, 100*(5), 1468–1481.

Center for Medicare and Medicaid Services. (2017). *Racial and ethnic disparities by gender in health care in Medicare Advantage*. Baltimore, MD: CMS Office of Minority Health and RAND Corporation. Retrieved from www.cms.gov/About-CMS/Agency-Information/OMH/Downloads/Health-Disparities-Racial-and-Ethnic-Disparities-by-Gender-National-Report.pdf

Cunningham, W. A., Johnson, M. K., Raye, C. L., Gatenby, J. C., Gore, J. C., & Banaji, M. R. (2004). Separable neural components in the processing of black and white faces. *Psychological Science, 15*(12), 806–813.

Dasgupta, N. (2013). Implicit attitudes and beliefs adapt to situations: A decade of research on the malleability of implicit prejudice, stereotypes, and the self-concept. *Advances in Experimental Social Psychology, 47*, 233–279.

Dehon, E., Weiss, N., Jones, J., Gaulconer, W., Hinton, E., & Sterling, S. (2017). A systematic review of the impact of physician implicit racial bias on clinical decision making. *Academic Emergency Medicine, 24*, 895–904.

Dreyer, R. P., Beltrame, J. F., Tavella, R., Air, T., Hoffmann, B., Pati, P. K., Di Fiore, D., Arstall, M., & Zeitz, C. (2013). Evaluation of gender differences in door-to-balloon time in ST-elevation myocardial infarction. *Heart, Lung and Circulation, 22*, 861–869.

Grant, J. M., Mottet, L. A., Tanis, J., Herman, J. L., Harrison, J., & Keisling, M. (2010). *National transgender discrimination survey report on health and health care.* National Center for Transgender Equality and National Gay and Lesbian Task Force. Retrieved from www.thetaskforce.org/static_html/downloads/resources_and_tools/ntds_report_on_health.pdf

Green, A. R., Carney, D. R., Pallin, D. J., Ngo, L. H., Raymond, K. L., & Iezzoni, L. I. (2007). Implicit bias among physicians and its prediction of thrombolysis decisions for black and white patients. *Journal of General Internal Medicine, 22*(9), 1231–1238.

Greenwald, A. G., McGhee, D. E., & Schwartz, J. L. K. (1998). Measuring individual differences in implicit cognition: The Implicit Association Test. *Journal of Personality and Social Psychology, 74*(6), 1464–1480.

Greenwald, A. G., Poehlman, T. A., Uhlmann, E. L., & Banaji, M. R. (2009). Understanding and using the Implicit Association Test: III. Meta-analysis of predictive validity. *Journal of Personality and Social Psychology, 97*(1), 17–41.

Haider, A. H., Schneider, E. B., Sriram, N., Scott, V. K., Swoboda, S. M., Zogg, C. K., . . . Cooper, L. A. (2015). Unconscious race and class biases among registered nurses: Vignette-based study using Implicit Association Testing. *Journal of the American College of Surgeons, 220*(6), 1077–1086.

Hamilton, S., Lewis-Holmes, E., Pinfold, V., Henderson, C., Rose, D., & Thornicroft, G. (2014). Discrimination against people with a mental health diagnosis: Qualitative analysis of reported experiences. *Journal of Mental Health, 23*(2), 88–93.

Hansson, L., Jormfeldt, H., Svedberg, P., & Svensson, B. (2011). Mental health professionals' attitudes towards people with mental illness: Do they differ from attitudes held by people with mental illness? *International Journal of Social Psychiatry, 59*(1), 48–54.

Harvey, V. L., & Housel, T. H. (Eds.). (2014). *Health care disparities and the LGBT population.* Lanham, MD: Lexington Books.

Healthy People 2020. (2018). *Lesbian, gay, bisexual, and transgender health.* Office of Health Promotion and Disease Prevention. Retrieved from www.healthypeople.gov/2020/topics-objectives/topic/lesbian-gay-bisexual-and-transgender-health/objectives

Human Rights Campaign. (n.d.). *Healthcare equality index.* Author. Retrieved from www.hrc.org/hei

Institute of Medicine. (2011). *The health of lesbian, gay, bisexual, and transgender people: Building a foundation for better understanding.* Washington, DC: National Academies.

James, S. E., Herman, J. L., Rankin, S., Keisling, M., Mottet, L., & Anafi, M. (2016). *The report of the 2015 U.S. transgender survey.* Washington, DC: National Center for Transgender Equality.

Jamieson, L. (2014, Spring). Grand unified theory of female pain. *Virginia Quarterly Review,* 114–128.

Kang, J. (2012). Communications law: Bits of bias. In J. D. Levinson & R. J. Smith (Eds.), *Implicit racial bias across the law.* New York: Cambridge University Press.

Kang, Y., Grey, J. R., Dovidio, J. F. (2014). The nondiscriminating heart: Lovingkindness meditation training decreases implicit intergroup bias. *Journal of Experimental Psychology, 143*(3), 1306–1313.

Kang, J., & Lane, K. (2010). Seeing through colorblindness: Implicit bias and the law. *UCLA Law Review, 58*(2), 465–520.

Kessler, R., Aguilar-Gaxiola, S., Alonso, J., Chatterji, S., Sing, L., Ormel, J., Ustun, T. B., & Wang, P. S. (2009). The global burden of mental disorders: An update from the WHO World Mental Health Surveys. *Epidemiologia e psichiatria sociale, 18*(1), 23–33.

Kisely, S., Sadek, J., MacKenzie, A., Lawrence, D., & Campbell, L. A. (2008). Excess cancer mortality in psychiatric patients. *Canadian Journal of Psychiatry, 53,* 753–761.

Laursen, T. M., Munk-Olsen, T., & Gasse, C. (2011). Chronic somatic comorbidity and excess mortality due to natural causes in persons with schizophrenia or bipolar affective disorder. *PLoS One, 6*(9), e24597. doi:10.1371/journal.pone.0024597

Laursen, T. M., Munk-Olsen, T., Nordentoft, M., & Mortensen, P. B. (2007). Increased mortality among patients admitted with major psychiatric disorders: A register-based study comparing mortality in unipolar depressive disorder, bipolar affective disorder, schizoaffective disorder, and schizophrenia. *Journal of Clinical Psychiatry, 68,* 899–907.

Laursen, T. M., Nordentoft, M., & Mortensen, P. B. (2014). Excess early mortality in schizophrenia. *Annual Review of Clinical Psychology, 10,* 425–448. doi:10.1146/annurev-clinpsy-032813-153657

Lieberman, M. D., Hariri, A., Jarcho, J. M., Eisenberger, N. I., & Bookheimer, S. Y. (2005). An fMRI investigation of race-related amygdala activity in African-American and Caucasian-American individuals. *Nature Neuroscience, 8*(6), 720–722.

Lorde, A. (1997). *The cancer journals, special edition.* San Francisco, CA: Aunt Lute Books.

Lueke, A., & Gibson, B. (2015). Mindfulness meditation reduces implicit age and race bias: The role of reduced automaticity of responding. *Social Psychological and Personality Science, 6*(3), 284–291.

Maserejian, N. N., Link, C., Lutfey, K. L., Marceau, L. D., & McKinlay, J. B. (2009). Disparities in physicians' interpretations of heart disease symptoms by patient gender: Results of a video vignette factorial experiment. *Journal of Women's Health, 18*(10), 1161–1667.

Maslow, A. H. (1966). *The psychology of science: A reconnaissance.* New York: Harper and Row.

Ottaway, S. A., Hayden, D. C., & Oakes, M. A. (2001). Implicit attitudes and racism: Effects of word familiarity and frequency on the Implicit Association Test. *Social Cognition, 19,* 97–144.

Phelan, S. M., Burgess, D. J., Yeazel, M. W., Hellerstedt, W. L., Griffin, J. M., & van Ryn, M. (2015). Impact of weight bias and stigma on quality of care and outcomes for patients with obesity. *Obesity Reviews, 16*(4), 319–326.

Phelps, E. A., O'Connor, K. J., Cunningham, W. A., Funayama, E. S., Gatenby, J. C., & Gore, J. C. (2000). Performance of indirect measures of race evaluation predicts amygdala activation. *Journal of Cognitive Neuroscience, 12*(5), 729–738.

Pierik, J. G. J, IJzerman, M. J., Gaakeer, M. I., Vollenbroek-Hutten, M. M. R., & Doggen, C. J. M. (2017). Painful discrimination in the emergency department: Risk factors for underassessment of patients' pain by nurses. *Journal of Emergency Nursing, 43,* 228–238.

Reskin, B. (2005). Unconsciousness raising. *Regional Review, 14*(3), 32–37.

Rudman, L. A. (2004). Social justice in our minds, homes, and society: The nature, causes, and consequences of implicit bias. *Social Justice Research, 17*(2), 129–142.

Sabin, J. A., & Greenwald, A. G. (2012). The influence of implicit bias on treatment recommendations for 4 common pediatric conditions: Pain, urinary tract infection, attention deficit hyperactivity disorder, and asthma. *American Journal of Public Health, 102*(5), 988–995.

Sabin, J. A., Nosek, B. A., Greenwald, A. G., & Rivara, F. P. (2009). Physicians' implicit and explicit attitudes about race by MD race, ethnicity, and gender. *Journal of Health Care for the Poor and Underserved, 20*(3), 896–913.

Shavers, V. L., Bakos, A., & Sheppard, V. B. (2010). Race, ethnicity, and pain among the U.S. adult population. *Journal of Health Care for the Poor and Underserved, 21*(1), 177–220.

Shefer, G., Henderson, C., Howard, L. M., Murray, J., & Thornicroft, G. (2014). Diagnostic overshadowing and other challenges involved in the diagnostic process of patients with mental illness who present in emergency departments with physical symptoms – A qualitative study. *PLoS One, 9*(11), e111682. doi:10.1371/journal. pone.0111682

Smedley, B. D., Stith, A. Y., & Nelson, A. R. (Eds.). (2003). *Unequal treatment: Confronting racial and ethnic disparities in health care.* Washington, DC: National Academies.

Society for Women's Health Research. (2017). Author. Retrieved from http://swhr. org/

Staats, C. (2014). *State of the science: Implicit bias review 2014.* Kirwan Institute for the Study of Race and Ethnicity. Retrieved from www.KirwanInstitute.osu.edu

Staats, C., Capatosto, K., Wright, R. A., & Jackson, V. W. (2016). *State of the science: Implicit bias review 2016.* Kirwan Institute for the Study of Race and Ethnicity. Retrieved from www.KirwanInstitute.osu.edu

Stell, A. J., & Farsides, T. (2016). Brief loving-kindness meditation reduces racial bias, mediated by positive other-regarding emotions. *Motivation and Emotion, 40*(1), 140–147.

Thornicroft, G. (2006). *Shunned: Discrimination against people with mental illness.* Oxford: Oxford University Press.

Thornicroft, G., Rose, D., & Kassam, A. (2007). Discrimination in health care against people with mental illness. *International Review of Psychiatry, 19*(2), 113–122.

Vanman, E. J., Saltz, J. L., Nathan, L. R., & Warren, J. A. (2004). Racial discrimination by low-prejudiced whites: Facial movements as implicit measures of attitudes related to behavior. *Psychological Science, 15*(11), 711–714.

World Health Organization. (2011). *Global burden of mental disorders and the need for a comprehensive, coordinated response from health and social sectors at the country level: Report from the secretariat.* Author. Retrieved from http://apps.who.int/gb/ebwha/pdf_files/EB130/B130_9-en.pdf

World Health Organization. (2013). *Mental health action plan 2013–2020.* Author. Retrieved from www.who.int/mental_health/publications/action_plan/en/

4 BEARING WITNESS TO SUFFERING

INTEGRATION NOTE

....

This chapter integrates with material on health professional well-being. The end-of-chapter activity aligns with clinical science education related to traumatic injury and disability studies.

INTRODUCTION

As health professionals, we spend our workday with people who are suffering from physical, emotional, social, spiritual, and economic burdens. Day after day, we care for people who struggle to breathe, writhe in pain, pray for mercy, endure abandonment, grapple with traumatic memories, dread the future, feel betrayed by their own bodies, grieve the loss of their identity and functionality, dodge abusive family members, and scrape to pay for food and medicine. Very early in our training, our innocence is stripped away. Human vulnerability is not an abstract concept to us – we see, hear, smell, and touch our patients' despair and frailty. Life is hard for many people, and made harder when coupled with disease. Whether consciously or not, when we decide to be health professionals, we sign up to come face to face with human suffering.

Health professionals bear witness to suffering – not as a matter of choice, but rather as a matter of circumstance. When we accept this circumstance, we can ready ourselves to understand suffering and recognize what happens when we are exposed regularly to suffering. The French philosopher, Jacques Derrida (2005, p. 82), writes,

> What distinguishes an act of bearing witness from the simple transmission of knowledge, from simple information, from the simple statement or mere demonstration of a proven theoretical truth, is that in it someone engages himself with regard to someone else.

Engagement is at the heart of the health professional–patient relationship, and engagement is a salve for the isolation that can accompany and magnify illness. When we witness and engage compassionately, we pierce our patients' isolation and offer the opportunity for transformation, growth, and healing – regardless of the prognosis – for the patient and ourselves. This is not an easy process. Our reflexive tendency may be to protect ourselves, to guard against the pain, and yet our professional calling is for compassionate engagement. How do we practice our profession, bear witness to suffering, compassionately engage with our patients, and not simply survive but thrive?

In this chapter, I present some introductory ideas about the philosophy of suffering from Western and Buddhist perspectives, and apply these perspectives to bearing witness in the clinical setting. I include the latest research about the potential negative effects bearing witness can have on health professionals in the form of compassion fatigue and vicarious trauma. Part of our professional development is learning to cope, in a healthy, nurturing way, with the emotions that arise when we bear witness to anguish, despair, pain, and sorrow. To that end, I describe effective interventions to mitigate the expense of bearing witness to our patients' suffering. The chapter concludes with exercises which actively engage the reader in the experience of bearing witness to suffering.

PHILOSOPHY OF SUFFERING

CULTURAL AND RELIGIOUS LENS

Those of us raised within a cultural or religious environment tend to be versed in the teachings of that environment, and will likely view this chapter through that lens. I encourage you to bring your cultural and religious beliefs about suffering to the fore of your consciousness and to use the contents of this chapter to tune those beliefs to focus on suffering in the context of clinical care. Although cultural and religious interpretations of suffering are beyond the scope of this chapter, they are integral to your personal development and self-care. Therefore, it is important that you consciously activate and use your cultural and religious beliefs as foundational material with which you assimilate the clinical context presented here. For example, if you have studied Judaism, Christianity, and/or Islam, then you probably learned about suffering from the Book of Job. Religious scholars and followers have interpreted Job's complex story myriad ways in an attempt to define why bad things happen to good people. Debate and controversy persist around the origin of suffering and the influence of evil. It is likely that at some point in your religious education, you made a decision about how to interpret Job's story for your personal life. This chapter does not intend to alter your interpretation, but rather aspires to broaden your thinking to include the suffering we see every day in clinical practice. That said, the remainder of this section will exclude religious references and will focus on secular views of suffering from Western and Buddhist philosophy.

DISTINCTION BETWEEN PAIN AND SUFFERING

At the outset, let's distinguish between pain and suffering. Although the words are semantically interchangeable in common parlance, pain and suffering are phenomenologically different (Casell, 2004). According to the International Association for the Study of Pain (2017), pain is "an unpleasant sensory and emotional experience associated with actual or potential tissue damage, or described in terms of such damage."

Suffering encompasses not only pain (physical and psychological), but also anguish, despair, grief, and a host of other responses that lead to existential crisis, "anything that threatens our personhood, our basic integrity, or intactness as existing individuals" (Madison, 2009, p. 8).

Many schools of philosophy have explored suffering and offered perspective on its relevance in human life. The scholarship is voluminous. For this chapter, I focus on philosophical reflections and arguments about the meaning of suffering and the transformation that can arise from suffering. The philosophy of suffering provides foundational material for our discussion, later in the chapter, about the effect on health professionals who bear witness to suffering.

WESTERN PHILOSOPHY

The ancient Stoic philosophers assert the basis for suffering is the judgment one makes of one's circumstance. If we ascertain a situation to be a threat to our self-identity and existence, then we suffer. If we ascertain the same situation to be painful but surmountable, then we endure the pain, but we do not suffer. The judgment we make, or more specifically, our interpretation of our life situation, then in turn offers us a remedy for our suffering since it "is the means whereby blind fate can be either the source of one's undoing or the means by which it can be transformed into a meaning-giving, life-enhancing challenge" (Madison, 2009, p. 9). If within the midst of our suffering, we can use our tragic circumstance as a crucible for awakening, then we have an opportunity to find meaning.

Miguel de Unamuno (1954, p. 140), Basque philosopher and professor, writes in his text, *The Tragic Sense of Life*, "Suffering is the path of consciousness, and by it living beings arrive at the possession of self-consciousness." Professor de Unamuno asserts that we must attain a sense of self in order to appreciate our distinction from others. Suffering makes us acutely aware of the limits of our being, "the point at which I cease to be" (p. 140). In this state of suffering we are truly aware that we exist, and thus become capable of igniting our empathic imagination to hear, see, and feel the plight of other living beings. By having an authentic, clear-eyed, undistracted experience of our own suffering, we are able to increase our conscious awareness of others' suffering. When we are aware that others are suffering, we cultivate our capacity for compassion.

While Professor de Unamuno sees suffering as a conduit for the sufferer to cultivate compassion, French philosopher, Emmanuel Levinas, offers a different perspective. Levinas (1987) perceives suffering as a state of humility wrought with awareness of one's tenuous claim to life. It is a state of unpretentious vulnerability, recognition of powerlessness to assert one's will, and termination of one's sense of self-mastery. In this humbled state, the sufferer requires "the Other" – the witness – to respond.

> In this perspective a radical difference develops between *suffering in the other*, which for *me* is unpardonable and solicits me and calls me, and suffering *in me*, my

own adventure of suffering, whose constitutional or congenital uselessness can take on a meaning, with only meaning to which suffering is susceptible, in becoming a suffering for the suffering – be it inexorable – of someone else.

(Levinas, 1988, p. 159) [italics in original text]

In brief, Levinas argues that suffering has meaning in that it demands a response from those who witness suffering. The witness has a responsibility to the sufferer and an obligation to carry out the "supreme ethical principle" (p. 159) to serve the sufferer. Levinas does not view the witness as necessarily motivated by compassion for the sufferer, but rather as having an obligation to the sufferer, regardless of impetus or feelings. Levinas acknowledges that serving the sufferer out of obligation can lead to resentment and moral anguish, and yet he remains committed to his assertion that suffering only has meaning when it stimulates the witness to act (White, 2012).

With the arguments of these Western philosophers in mind, let's turn our attention to Buddhist philosophy.

BUDDHIST PHILOSOPHY

Within the major Buddhist schools of thought, Theravada, Indian Mahayana, Tibetan Mahayana and Vajrayana, and East Asian Buddhism, there are a wealth of teachings about suffering (Emmanuel, 2013). The conceptual foundations common among the schools are the Four Noble Truths, stated here:

(i) dukka, "the painful," encompassing the various forms of "pain," gross or subtle, physical or mental, to which we are all subject, along with painful things that engender these; (ii) the origination (samudaya, i.e., cause) of dukkha, namely craving; (iii) the cessation (nirodha) of dukkha by the cessation of craving (this cessation being equivalent to nirvana); and (iv) the Noble Eight-Factored Path (magga) that leads to this cessation.

(p. 62)

Author, peace activist, and Zen Buddhist master teacher, Thich Nhat Hanh (2014, p. 11), interprets the Four Noble Truths for Western readers in his text, *No Mud, No Lotus: The Art of Transforming Suffering*.

The very first teaching the Buddha gave after his enlightenment was about suffering. . . . The Buddha's Four Noble Truths are: there is suffering; there is a course of action that generates suffering; suffering ceases (i.e., there is happiness); and there is a course of action leading to the cessation of suffering (the arising of happiness).

Thich Nhat Hanh goes on to describe transformation that may come from suffering.

When you first hear that suffering is a Noble Truth, you might wonder what's so noble about suffering? The Buddha was saying that if we can recognize suffering, and if we embrace it and look deeply into its roots, then we'll be able to let go of the habits that feed it and, at the same time, find a way to happiness. Suffering has its beneficial aspects. It can be an excellent teacher.

In the clinical setting, the Four Noble Truths have relevance to both the sufferer (patient) and the witness (health professional). Once we acknowledge that suffering is an essential component of happiness – in the same way that there is no light without darkness nor left without right – then our attention can turn away from despair and toward reestablishing equanimity. Buddhist philosophy takes us beyond Western arguments for using suffering to awaken our compassion or fulfill our responsibility and obligation, to a state of deep understanding and intimacy with the nature of our personal causative agents for suffering. In this state of deep understanding, we are liberated to act with mindful awareness and compassion, which is Buddhism's purported pathway to suffer less (Rahula, 2018).

HEALTH PROFESSIONALS' EXPERIENCES OF BEARING WITNESS TO SUFFERING

Although philosophical perspectives, as previously described, offer us an opportunity to find meaning in suffering, health professionals rarely have the opportunity to explore or apply philosophical arguments in the clinical setting. In the past few years, an increasing number of health professionals have written about their experience of bearing witness to their patients' suffering. Accounts of the negative effects of bearing witness to suffering far outweigh reports of transformational growth. In the comprehensive text, *The Nature of Suffering and the Goals of Nursing*, Betty Ferrell and Nessa Coyle (2014) offer compelling accounts of suffering by patients, their family members, and the nurses who care for them. As reported by Ferrell and Coyle, nurses who bear witness to patients' suffering often express moral distress and anger at having to provide futile care, anguish at having to cause pain during the course of care and at prolonging the dying process, and angst that they are not respected or heard by other members of the healthcare team. In summarizing their interviews with nurses, Ferrell and Coyle excerpt the nurses' words in this quote: "The words . . . illustrate the powerful emotions of nurses as they describe 'violent acts,' 'torture,' and feeling 'disempowered'" (p. 91). This is in contradistinction to nurses who describe their work as "sacred care" when they are able to be fully present and aware of their patient's "deep and profound experience of suffering" (p. 5).

University of Zurich nurse researcher, Rahel Naef, RN, PhD, offers a convincing philosophical argument for nurses' moral responsibility to bear witness to patients. Naef (2006, p. 149) writes,

we can choose to bear witness to the other's vulnerability or we can refuse to bear witness. However, we cannot escape the responsibility, but paradoxically, we can negate the other by turning away and leaving him or her deserted in his or her aloneness and suffering. We can respect, revere, and honour the other's humanity, or we can leave him or her in total isolation, negating his or her existence as a human being, including the need for recognition and human connectedness.

Instead of describing the burden of bearing witness, Naef (2006, p. 152) describes the consequences of *not* bearing witness, of "turning away."

> Experiences and situations where we turn away, or where we are unable to bear witness for whatever reasons can become stories that haunt us. They become stories of constrained moral agency.

Naef provides a rare pivot in orientation. As you'll see later in this chapter, there is a deep literature that explores the burden of bearing witness (see Effects of Witnessing on Health Professionals section). In contrast, Naef demands that we think about what happens when we dismiss our moral responsibility to bear witness to our patients' suffering. When we turn away and negate our patients' personhood, we simultaneously negate our own humanity.

Writer and physician, Rose Kumar, MD (2013), invokes transcendent language when describing her experience of bearing witness to patients' suffering.

> As a physician, I feel that bearing witness is the most sacred part of what I do each day. Holding space and bearing witness to sometimes unbearable suffering deepens my heart and fortifies my soul. It makes my patients feel that they matter, that their pain and suffering matters. To be asked to bear witness for another is a profound honor.

Physician John Schumann, MD discloses that it took him a number of years in clinical practice to recognize the value and privilege of bearing witness to patients. He had to grapple with medicine's limitations, wrestle with uncertainty as an inherent component of patient care, and strive to understand his patients' perspectives on illness before he allowed himself to know the merits of bearing witness. Dr. Schumann (2013) writes, "Bearing witness is incredibly powerful. Listening to others share their stories of illness and suffering is enriching – for the subject and the listener."

EFFECTS OF WITNESSING ON HEALTH PROFESSIONALS

It is essential that we approach our role of witness to our patients' suffering with thought, care, and intention; otherwise, it is easy for us to fall prey to the negative effects of witnessing. Over the past couple of decades, an emerging literature has investigated the constructs of compassion fatigue, vicarious trauma, and related entities. These constructs aim to capture the occupational hazards faced by health professionals (and other service professionals) who have repeated exposure to the suffering of others. Literature reviews confirm a variety of definitions for compassion fatigue and vicarious trauma in use among researchers (Ledoux, 2015; Najjar, Davis, Beck-Coon, & Doebbeling, 2009). There appears to be considerable conflation among compassion fatigue, vicarious trauma, and burnout, with no clear, universally accepted distinctive criteria. All three constructs may lead to physical and emotional exhaustion, disengagement from work, and emotional distancing from patients, colleagues, friends, and family. The lack of a uniform taxonomy seriously undermines advancement of the field and prevents precise estimates of prevalence (van Mol, Kompanje, Benoit, Bakker, & Nijkamp, 2015). For the purpose of this chapter, we need to understand that health professionals potentially incur harm from bearing witness – regardless of whether we label the harm compassion fatigue, vicarious trauma, burnout, or something else. I provide working definitions of compassion fatigue and vicarious trauma, since they appear to be phenomenologically different, particularly in derivation if not in expression. I also highlight some of the research that explores each construct among health professionals. I defer in-depth discussion of burnout until chapter 5 Resilience and Burnout.

For research to advance understanding of the effects of bearing witness to suffering for health professionals, we need to assure standardization of taxonomy and metrics. There also needs to be clarity about the physiologic and behavioral links between empathy, compassion, and vulnerability with outcomes such as compassion fatigue, vicarious trauma, and burnout. I encourage the interested reader to consider contributing to this nascent field of research.

COMPASSION FATIGUE

Nurse researcher Carla Joinson (1992) first described compassion fatigue in 1992 when studying burnout in emergency department nurses. Psychologist Charles Figley (2002, p. 1435) proposed a formal definition,

> a state of tension and preoccupation with the traumatized patients by re-experiencing the traumatic events, avoidance/numbing of reminders, persistent arousal (e.g., anxiety) associated with the patient. It is a function of bearing witness to the suffering of others.

Building on Figley's work, psychologist Beth Stamm proposed the Theoretical Model of Compassion Satisfaction and Compassion Fatigue, which relates the positive and negative aspects of work for service professionals. The model purports compassion fatigue is comprised of burnout (exhaustion, frustration, anger, depression, distress by work environment) and secondary traumatic stress, "a negative feeling driven by fear and work-related trauma" (Stamm, 2010).

RESEARCH STUDIES OF COMPASSION FATIGUE AMONG HEALTH PROFESSIONALS

Qualitative phenomenological interviews with registered nurses working at a level-1 trauma center in the United States demonstrate the Theoretical Model of Compassion

Satisfaction and Compassion Fatigue (described earlier) may not sufficiently characterize the experience of nurses. The author reports the emergence of four additional themes from the interviews, including: "belief in the unfairness of life, feeling saturated by emotions, being unable to disconnect when away from work, and wanting support but pushing away" (Sheppard, 2015, p. 58).

A 2013 survey study in Israel used a national sample of mental health and medical practitioners to identify personal factors predictive of compassion fatigue (Zeidner, Hadar, Matthews, & Roberts, 2013). The study results showed emotional intelligence, emotion management, and adaptive coping style related inversely to compassion fatigue. This means that among the mental health and medical practitioners in the study, those who were highly capable of perceiving and understanding emotions in oneself and others, accessing and generating emotions, as well as reflectively regulating emotions, were less likely to experience compassion fatigue than those who did not have these qualities of emotional intelligence and emotion management. Similarly, participants who reported an adaptive coping style, which customarily focuses on problem solving, were less likely to experience compassion fatigue than those who reported emotion-focused and avoidance coping styles. Of note, there were no significant group differences in compassion fatigue between the mental health practitioners and the medical practitioners; and there were no significant differences by gender for compassion fatigue.

BOX 4.1 THICH NHAT HANH AND COMPASSION FATIGUE

In 2011, I attended a retreat led by author, peace activist, and Zen Buddhist master teacher, Thich Nhat Hanh, at Blue Cliff Monastery in New York. After Thich Nhat Hanh shared a profound teaching about cultivating compassion for self and others, one of the retreatants asked him how to protect herself from compassion fatigue. Thich Nhat Hanh was puzzled by the phrase compassion fatigue. He asked the retreatant to explain the phrase. The retreatant talked about feeling exhausted from caring too much and losing her sense of self from excessive engagement with patients. In his kind, gentle, and fierce way, Thich Nhat Hanh explained that compassion is an indefatigable wellspring. Compassion yields more compassion. It is inherently salubrious, and thereby energizing – never fatiguing. When we find ourselves depleted, exhausted, fearful, and alienated, it is not from caring too much. It may be that we have not given proper attention to our own suffering such that when we are exposed to another person's suffering our own issues become inflamed. Thich Nhat Hanh recommends applying mindfulness training (see chapter 6 Recognizing Our Interdependence, the Mindfulness section), looking deeply within, acknowledging the pain that has come to us and that we have generated, and offering love and compassion to ourselves.

VICARIOUS TRAUMA

Vicarious trauma was first described by psychologists Lisa McCann and Laurie Anne Pearlman (1990) who positioned vicarious trauma as a unique phenomenon of trauma workers who internalize but do not sufficiently process the horrors, atrocities, and suffering experienced by their clients and patients. Using research from professionals who worked with Holocaust survivors and Vietnam War veterans, McCann and Pearlman originally grounded vicarious trauma in a model of countertransference; however, later publications diminished the influence of the health professional's personal history. Although often used interchangeably with compassion fatigue, secondary traumatic stress, and burnout, the definition here indicates criteria exclusive to vicarious trauma: "negative transformation in the self of a trauma worker or helper that results from empathic engagement with traumatized clients and their reports of traumatic experiences. Its hallmark is disrupted spirituality or meaning and hope" (Pearlman, 2012, p. 783). Vicarious trauma fundamentally differs from compassion fatigue in that vicarious trauma is founded in theory (namely, constructivist self-development theory) rather than simply being an observable constellation of symptoms. Similar to compassion fatigue and burnout, the health professional who experiences vicarious trauma may have physical and emotional exhaustion. Vicarious trauma, however, is distinct in that it specifically includes trauma-specific symptoms, such as intrusive imagery, that are not customarily a part of compassion fatigue and burnout.

> Common signs and symptoms include, but are not limited to, social withdrawal, emotional dysregulation, aggression, greater sensitivity to violence, somatic symptoms, sleep difficulties, intrusive imagery, cynicism, anxiety, depression, substance overuse, sexual difficulties, difficulty managing boundaries with clients, and disruptions in core beliefs and resulting difficulty in relationships reflecting problems with security, trust, esteem, intimacy, and control.
>
> (Pearlman, 2012, p. 783)

RESEARCH STUDY OF VICARIOUS TRAUMA AMONG HEALTH PROFESSIONALS

The literature is comprised predominantly of research about mental health workers, especially those who care for victims of sexual assault, other interpersonal violence, including war crimes, and natural disasters. More recently, there has been an effort to include physicians, nurses, and other health professionals who work in emergency medicine, critical care, and elsewhere in the tertiary care environment. A 2013 study evaluated physicians and nurses working in hospitals in Iasi, Romania to identify predictive factors for vicarious trauma (Mairean & Turliuc, 2013). Participants were assessed for personality trait (openness to new experiences, conscientiousness, extraversion, agreeableness, and neuroticism), coping orientation (problem-focused, emotion-focused, and dysfunctional coping), direct and indirect experiences of trauma, and vicarious trauma beliefs, which are cognitive changes resulting from secondary exposure to trauma. Multiple regression analysis showed neuroticism personality trait was a positive predictor of vicarious trauma beliefs, while extraversion and conscientiousness personality traits negatively, or inversely, predicted vicarious trauma beliefs. A form of emotion-focused coping, positive reinterpretation, also inversely predicted vicarious trauma beliefs. Personality trait accounted for 36% of variation, and coping orientation accounted for 39% of variation in vicarious trauma beliefs. The study limitations include exclusive reliance on participants' self-reports and historical recall of coping efforts. That said, the study demonstrated considerable interplay among personality trait, coping orientation, and vicarious trauma beliefs that warrants further investigation.

BIOLOGICAL MECHANISMS OF COMPASSION AND EMPATHY

There is ongoing effort in multiple disciplines to identify the biological mechanisms of compassion and empathy. At present, controversy and debate prevail over unified theory. That said, it is worth recounting peak areas of inquiry here. A recent article by Mark Russell and Matt Brickell (2015) provides an overview of the working neurobehavioral theories of compassion stress. Russell and Brickell report on the convergence of neuroscientific models that assert empathy is generated by two parallel processes, one non-conscious and one conscious. Non-conscious or automatic process pairs perception and action. It is the initial empathic response triggered by activation of "mirroring neural circuits involved in imitation, mimicry, and emotional contagion, all outside the observer's conscious awareness or control" (p. 1097). Conscious (or cognitively controlled) process acts to regulate self/other awareness, perspective-taking, the empathic response, and prosocial, altruistic behavior.

While still a burgeoning field of inquiry, the neuroscientific models show increasing evidence for a biological mechanism of compassion and empathy. When neuroscience research is coupled with psycho-behavioral research, there is compelling trend data to indicate effective interventions for health professionals to mitigate the expense of bearing witness to suffering and, potentially, undergo transformational growth (Pearlman, 2012).

EFFECTIVE INTERVENTIONS TO MITIGATE THE EXPENSE OF BEARING WITNESS

Presented here are interventions that have demonstrated effectiveness in helping people bear witness.

SELF-AWARENESS

The first and vital step to mitigate the expense of bearing witness to suffering is to know one's self. We each need to invest time developing our self-awareness so we know our own stored suffering and the external circumstances that make us react. Equipped with self-knowledge, we can proactively prevent spiraling into a state of reactivity fueled largely by our unconscious mind. Getting to know one's self takes time and concerted effort; however, the rewards to one's self and others are immeasurable. The topic of self-awareness is visited additionally in chapter 3 Unconscious Bias.

CONTEMPLATIVE PRACTICE

Contemplative practices are one of many pathways to increase self-awareness. Contemplative practices, both religious and secular, offer the opportunity to develop discriminating focused attention and concentration on our thoughts, emotions, behaviors, and beliefs. With objective, non-judgmental discernment, we come to understand what gives our life meaning, purpose, and value, as well as what keeps us trapped in habitual patterns of reactivity. Often, contemplative practices help us to see the vestiges of past wounds, regrets, grief, and anguish that lie hidden from our everyday attention and yet feed our unconscious mind with bitterness, cynicism, anxiety, and sadness. Once we are aware of these hidden parts of ourselves, then we can consciously work to reclaim their potency for transformational growth.

I encourage you to find a contemplative practice that resonates with your core beliefs and nature. If you have a religious affiliation, you may want to explore the contemplative arm of your faith tradition. Readers with a secular orientation may wish to explore meditation practices. The text, *Contemplative Practices in Action: Spirituality, Meditation, and Health,* provides an overview of several contemplative practices and may be a good place to start your investigation to promote self-awareness (Plante, 2010).

LOVING-KINDNESS MEDITATION

Surrounded by human tragedy on a regular basis, it is easy for health professionals to think of ourselves as pawns of the medical-industrial complex who patch up people so they can return to their lives, only to repeatedly cycle back for care. When we feel that our efforts are futile against the barrage of human suffering, it helps to remember that our presence, solid and sincere, is often powerful medicine. To bear the effects of witnessing suffering, we need to be tender and kind to ourselves.

Metta, or loving-kindness meditation, is a 5th-century C.E. practice rooted in the Theravada Buddhist traditions which helps us cultivate warmth, tenderness, and kindness toward ourselves and others (Nhat Hanh, 2010). Loving-kindness meditation is taught to health professionals enrolled in hospice and palliative care training at the Metta Institute and Upaya Zen Center, however, to date I have not seen published effectiveness studies. Based on my own experiences and those of colleagues, I recommend you experiment with this simple and profound practice. Following is a brief description of one of the loving-kindness practices.

Sharon Salzberg (2002), co-founder of the Insight Meditation Society, Buddhist meditation teacher, and author, presents a detailed and nuanced discussion of loving-kindness practice for Westerners in her book, *Lovingkindness: The Revolutionary Art of Happiness.* Ms. Salzberg shares several metta practices in her text. Here are her instructions for practicing loving-kindness toward one's self. Of note, practicing loving-kindness toward one's self is considered a first step before we offer loving-kindness to someone who has been kind to us, someone we feel neutral about (e.g., the postal carrier), someone we love, and someone who has caused us harm.

> Sit comfortably. You can begin with five minutes of reflection on the good within you or your wish to be happy. . . . Without trying to force or demand a loving feeling, see if there are circumstances you can imagine yourself in where you can more readily experience friendship with yourself
>
> Develop a gentle pacing with the phrases; there is no need to rush through them or say them harshly. You are offering yourself a gift with each phrase. If your attention wanders, or if difficult feelings or memories arise, try to let go of them in the spirit of kindness, and begin again repeating the metta phrases:
>
> > May I be free from danger.
> > May I have mental happiness.
> > May I have physical happiness.
> > May I have ease of well-being.
>
> There are times when feelings of unworthiness come up strongly, and you clearly see the conditions that limit your love for yourself. Breathe gently, accept that these feelings have arisen, remember the beauty of your wish to be happy, and return to the metta phrases.
>
> > > > > (p. 31)

SOCIAL SUPPORT

Social support can be a helpful intervention to mitigate the negative effects from bearing witness to suffering (Ariapooran, 2014; Michalopoulos & Aparicio, 2012). Having someone to talk to about the human devastation one sees, especially someone who has experienced your vantage point and shares your values – like a professional peer – can help you stay oriented and focused on finding meaning.

BALINT GROUPS

Balint groups are one such approach to supportive social processing for health professionals. Balint groups typically are led by a trained facilitator. One member of the group shares a story, without interruption, about a patient encounter. After a brief period clarifying facts, the storyteller sits back and listens without comment as the rest of the group discusses the story. The discussion is not about standards of care and interpreting diagnostic studies, but rather attends to the group members' reflections about the story, how they think the patient feels, what they think the patient wants from the encounter, and how they would feel if they were the health professional. The emphasis is on support, respect, and reflective inquiry into "the patient as a person and the emotional interaction" with the health professional (Salinsky, 2013).

A recent research study in Australia explored the effect of Balint groups on compassion fatigue and burnout experienced by physicians in obstetrics and gynecology who regularly care for patients who suffer traumatic birth and/or fetal demise, experience life-altering diagnoses and aggressive care, and/or live with complex psychosocial circumstances. Pre- and post-intervention surveys showed significantly lower levels of compassion fatigue and burnout among participants. In addition, results showed a significant increase in the number of participants who experienced compassion satisfaction (Allen, Watt, Jansen, Coghlan, & Nathan, 2017).

THE ARTS

Throughout history, humans have used the arts to express pain, sorrow, joy, misery, confusion, revelation, surrender, defiance, and more. Whether creating the artistic piece or reflecting upon it, art can awaken dormant feelings within us and bring us to a heightened state of awareness. Art forms – spoken word, written word, visual art, performance art, music – invite us to see the familiar in a new way, to reintroduce ourselves to our inner and outer world. Art historian Ernst Gombrich (1987, p. 211) writes,

> art is an institution to which we turn when we want to feel a shock of surprise. We feel this want because we sense that it is good for us once in a while to receive a healthy jolt. Otherwise we would so easily get stuck in a rut and could no longer adapt to the new demands that life is apt to make on us. The biological function of art, in other words, is that of a rehearsal, a training in mental gymnastics which increases our tolerance of the unexpected.

A 2018 survey study of United States medical students (N = 739) demonstrates significant direct correlations between exposure to the humanities (e.g., active and passive engagement with music, literature, theater, and/or visual arts) and positive qualities such as empathy, tolerance for ambiguity, and wisdom. In addition, exposure to the humanities was inversely correlated with indicators of burnout (Mangione et al., 2018). The authors conclude, "The humanities might actually provide an indispensable *language* for exploring that strange, nuanced, and often nonsensical land called the human condition" (p. 633, [italics in original text]).

Art gives us the potential to expand our vision such that it may be possible to see joy and beauty as companions to suffering, and allow meaning to emerge from despair. My personal experience with art forms that have magnified my perceptions include the musical composition, *Water from an Ancient Well*, by Abdullah Ibrahim (1986). Its melody evokes sorrow and longing, intermingled with hope – not naïve or innocent hope, but rather the hope that arises from love, respect, and faith in something greater than one's self. The plaintive call of *Water from an Ancient Well* arouses courage and optimism in me.

TELLING OUR STORIES

Reflecting on and writing our patient care stories can help us to drop our stoic bravado, recognize the burden we are carrying, and approach our pain with insight and authenticity. For many, writing our stories, making them external to our being, lightens our perceived load and allows us to reconnect with our core beliefs and find our purpose. Nellie Hermann (2017), in the text, *The Principals and Practices of Narrative Medicine*, describes three byproducts of writing our stories. By externalizing content we open up space for new experiences; we create a tangible product (the written piece) that can be explored; and (when we have a readership) we allow others to share in our experience, examine the content from their perspectives, and enliven us with their insights.

Social psychologist James Pennebaker has spent decades studying the health effects of expressive writing, a technique that has participants write for a brief period (15–20 minutes) each day for several consecutive days about their emotions and thoughts toward a personally traumatic or upsetting event. Hundreds of studies have used the expressive writing intervention with largely favorable results. There is evidence of physiologic benefit, in the form of improved immune function, as well as psychological benefit (Pennebaker & Smyth, 2016).

Medical sociologist, Arthur Frank, PhD (2013) writes in *The Wounded Storyteller* about the empathic bonds that stories create between the storyteller and the reader. Writing one's story is a way to recover one's voice and make familiar that which is egregious and alien. Writing contextualizes human suffering within the larger frame of the human condition, and allows the writer and reader to open to new perspectives and recognize the universality of the story.

In the text, *Privileged Presence: Personal Stories of Connection in Healthcare*, Liz Crocker and Bev Johnson have collected stories from patients, family members, and health professionals. Crocker and Johnson (2014, p. 310) write,

> Health care professionals, too, have stories to tell. These men and women keep company with suffering of others and walk with them through profound events. The world of health care professionals is full of long hours, pressured situations, hard work, miracles, and tragedies. It can be a raw place with its own pain, fear of the unknown, and loss of meaning. For health care professionals, too, then, telling their stories helps provide comfort and healing for the dramatic work they do. For all, telling stories helps provide meaning in chaos.

CLOSING

In this chapter, we looked at the philosophy of suffering from Western and Buddhist perspectives to provide a foundation for our discussion of health professionals bearing witness. We heard from health professionals about their experiences, positive and negative, of bearing witness to suffering. We reviewed some of the literature related to compassion fatigue and vicarious trauma, and then looked at ways to mitigate the negative effects of witnessing human suffering.

I close this chapter with learning objectives and activities that provide the reader with the personal experience of bearing witness to suffering while in a controlled setting. The learning activities allow you to observe your own reactions to suffering without the competing demands of providing care to a patient, thus making your experience a personal learning laboratory on bearing witness to suffering.

ACTIVITIES

LEARNING OBJECTIVES

Learners will

1 discuss the experience of bearing witness to another's suffering;
2 reflect on their personal experience of bearing witness.

PODCAST AND DISCUSSION

First, listen to the Snap Judgment podcast, *Falling Slowly* (Thau & Sussman, 2015). The podcast is available at http://snapjudgment.org/falling-slowly. As you read, note words or passages that appeal to you, repel you, resonate with you, startle you, or in some way catch your attention. Drawing on material presented in chapter 4, reflect on your personal experience of bearing witness to the suffering of Lee-Anna, the storyteller.

SMALL GROUP DISCUSSION

Learners are invited to discuss their experience with the podcast. Whenever possible, learners should refer to specific passages in the podcast. In particular, learners should aim to comment on their experience of bearing witness to Lee-Anna's suffering.

NOTE: **Appendix A** has general guidelines for facilitating a health humanities seminar. **Appendix B** has instruction and discussion prompts specific to this activity for faculty facilitators to use if your learners are not able to initiate a robust discussion.

WRITING AND SHARING

The second activity is for the learner to write to a prompt that directly links the chapter content and the podcast. Here is a suggested writing prompt:

> Write about a time you witnessed someone suffering. Feel free to write fiction.

Faculty facilitators can invite the learners to share what they have written with the group. Learners should never be required to share their writings.

REFERENCE LIST

Allen, R., Watt, F., Jansen, B., Coghlan, E., & Nathan, E. A. (2017). Minimising compassion fatigue in obstretrics/gynaecology doctors: Exploring an intervention for an occupational hazard. *Australasian Psychiatry, 25*(4), 403–406.

Ariapooran, S. (2014). Compassion fatigue and burnout in Iranian nurses: The role of perceived social support. *Iranian Journal of Nurse Midwifery Research, 19*(3), 279–284.

Casell, E. (2004). *The nature of suffering and the goals of medicine* (2nd ed.). New York: Oxford University Press.

Crocker, L., & Johnson, B. (2014). *Privileged presence: Personal stories of connection in healthcare* (2nd ed.). Boulder, CO: Bull.

de Unamuno, M. (1954). *Tragic sense of life*. Translated by J. E. Crawford Flitch. New York: Dover.

Derrida, J. (2005). Poetics and politics of witnessing. In T. Dutoit & O. Pasanen (Eds.), *Sovereignties in question: The poetics of Paul Celan*. New York: Fordham University.

Emmanuel, S. M. (Ed.). (2013). *A companion to Buddhist philosophy*. West Sussex, UK: Wiley-Blackwell.

Ferrell, B., & Coyle, N. (2014). *The nature of suffering and the goals of nursing*. New York: Oxford University Press.

Figley, C. R. (2002). Compassion fatigue: Psychotherapists' chronic lack of self care. *Journal of Clinical Psychology, 58*, 1433–1441.

Frank, A. (2013). *The wounded storyteller: Body, illness, and ethics* (2nd ed.). Chicago, IL: University of Chicago Press.

Gombrich, E. H. (1987). *Reflections on the history of art*. Berkeley, CA: University of California Press.

Hermann, N. (2017). Creativity. In R. Charon, S. Das Gupta, N. Hermann, C. Irvine, E. R. Marcus, E. Rivera Colon, D. Spencer, & M. Spiegel (Eds.), *The principles and practices of narrative medicine* (pp. 211–232). New York: Oxford University Press.

Ibrahim, A. (1986). Water from an ancient well. In *Water from an ancient well*. Frankfurt am Main: Bellaphon Records.

International Association for the Study of Pain. (2017). *IASP terminology: Pain*. Author. Retrieved from www.iasp-pain.org/Education/Content. aspx?ItemNumber=1698#Pain

Joinson, C. (1992). Coping with compassion fatigue. *Nursing, 22*, 116–121.

Kumar, R. (2013). The power of bearing witness. *Huffington Post*. Retrieved from www.huffingtonpost.com/rose-kumar-md/conscious-relationships_b_4333957.html

Ledoux, K. (2015). Understanding compassion fatigue: Understanding compassion. *Journal of Advanced Nursing, 71*(9), 2041–2050.

Levinas, E. (1987). *Time and the other*. Translated by R. Cohen. Pittsburgh, PA: Duquesne University.

Levinas, E. (1988). Useless suffering. In R. Bernasconi & D. Wood (Eds.), *The provocation of Levinas*. London: Routledge.

Madison, G. B. (2009). *On suffering: Philosophical reflections on what it means to be human*. Hamilton, Ontario, CA: Les Érables.

Mairean, C., & Turliuc, M. N. (2013). Predictors of vicarious trauma beliefs among medical staff. *Journal of Loss and Trauma, 18*, 414–428.

Mangione, S., Chakraborti, C., Staltari, G., Harrison, R., Tunkel, A. R., Liou, K. T., . . . Kahn, M. J. (2018). Medical students' exposure to the humanities correlates with positive personal qualities and reduced burnout: A multi-institutional US survey. *Journal of General Internal Medicine, 33*, 628–634, doi:10.1007/s11606-017-4275-8

McCann, I. L., & Pearlman, L. A. (1990). Vicarious traumatization: A framework for understanding the psychological effects of working with victims. *Journal of Traumatic Stress, 3*, 131–149.

Michalopoulos, L. M., & Aparicio, E. (2012). Vicarious trauma in social workers: The role of trauma history, social support, and years of experience. *Journal of Aggression, Maltreatment & Trauma, 21*, 646–664.

Naef, R. (2006). Bearing witness: A moral way of engaging in the nurse-person relationship. *Nursing Philosophy, 7*, 146–156.

Najjar, N., Davis, L. W., Beck-Coon, K., & Doebbeling, C. C. (2009). Compassion fatigue: A review of the research to date and relevance to cancer-care providers. *Journal of Health Psychology, 14*(2), 267–277.

Nhat Hanh, T. (2010). *Reconciliation: Healing the inner child*. Berkeley CA: Parallax.

Nhat Hanh, T. (2014). *No mud, no lotus: The art of transforming suffering*. Berkeley, CA: Parallax.

Pearlman, L. A. (2012). Vicarious trauma. In C. Figley (Ed.), *Encyclopedia of trauma: An interdisciplinary guide* (pp. 783–786). Thousand Oaks, CA: Sage.

Pennebaker, J. W., & Smyth, J. M. (2016). *Opening up by writing it down: How expressive writing improves health and eases emotional pain* (3rd ed.). New York and London: Guilford.

Plante, T. G. (Ed.). (2010). *Contemplative practices in action: Spirituality, meditation, and health*. Santa Barbara, CA: Praeger.

Rahula, W. (2018). The noble eightfold path: The Buddha's practical instructions to reach the end of suffering. *Tricycle Magazine*. Retrieved from https://tricycle.org/magazine/noble-eightfold-path/

Russell, M., & Brickell, M. (2015). The "double-edge sword" of human empathy: A unifying neurobehavioral theory of compassion stress injury. *Social Sciences, 4,* 1087–1117.

Salinsky, J. (2013). Balint groups and the Balint method. *The Balint Society*. Retrieved from https://balint.co.uk/about/the-balint-method/

Salzberg, S. (2002). *Lovingkindness: The revolutionary art of happiness*. Boston, MA and London: Shambala.

Schumann, J. (2013). Being a good doctor requires bearing witness. *Kevinmd.* Retrieved from www.kevinmd.com/blog/2013/09/good-doctor-requires-bearing-witness.html

Sheppard, K. (2015). Compassion fatigue among registered nurses: Connecting theory and research. *Applied Nursing Research, 28,* 57–59, doi:10.1016/j.apnr.2014.10.007

Stamm, B. H. (2010). *The concise ProQOL manual* (2nd ed.). ProQOL. Retrieved from www.ProQOL.org

Thau, L., & Sussman, A. (Producer) (2015). *Snap judgment: Falling slowly* [audio podcast]. Retrieved from http://snapjudgment.org/falling-slowly

van Mol, M. M. C., Kompanje, E. J. O., Benoit, D. D., Bakker, J., & Nijkamp, M. D. (2015). The prevalence of compassion fatigue and burnout among healthcare professionals in intensive care units: A systematic review. *PLoS One, 10*(8), e0136955. doi:10.1371/journal.pone.0136955

White, R. (2012). Levinas, the philosophy of suffering, and the ethics of compassion. *The Heythrop Journal, LIII*, 111–123.

Zeidner, M., Hadar, D., Matthews, G., & Roberts, R. D. (2013). Personal factors related to compassion fatigue in health professionals. *Anxiety, Stress, & Coping, 26*(6), 595–609.

5 RESILIENCE AND BURNOUT

INTEGRATION NOTE
....

This chapter integrates with health professional well-being education and content related to medical error. The learner activities at the end of the chapter align with curriculum content related to breast cancer and body image.

INTRODUCTION

When we are resilient, we are able to confidently rely on our preparation and aptitude to surmount the challenges we encounter. We uphold a broad vision such that we preserve a sense of beauty surrounding, and even permeating, the challenge and the scars it may leave behind. In contrast, if we have not cultivated resilience, we may become overwhelmed and experience distress and despair when faced with a challenge. Without resilience, we have a limited perception of our available resources and a very narrow view of possible solutions. Consequently, we may become defensive, apathetic, emotionally exhausted, and believe that our life has no purpose and our work is no longer meaningful – this is called burnout.

All of us, at some time in our lives, have faced a daunting challenge, be it a major injury or illness, the death of someone close to us, the demise of an intimate relationship, financial worries, physical or emotional assault, natural disaster, war, or professional burnout. Why is it that sometimes we respond successfully to a challenge and in turn grow stronger from the experience; whereas, at other times we succumb to despair? Researchers have devoted a great deal of attention to this question. We will delve into this research, particularly as it relates to health professionals.

In this chapter, I present some introductory material on biological and psychological features of resilience, and then compare resilience to burnout. I talk about the prevalence of burnout in the health professions and the staggering cost burnout exacts from individuals, families, and society. I explore research examining the protective factors that resilience offers against burnout in the context of healthcare and health professional education. I share ideas about interventions to help cultivate resilience for our personal well-being and so we can optimally serve others. I close the chapter with activities that provide opportunity for experiential learning related to cultivating resilience.

SCIENCE OF RESILIENCE

In this section, I provide a definition of resilience, briefly review salient scientific findings on resilience, and discuss recent research on toxic stress, changes in brain architecture, and epigenetic influences on resilience.

MULTIDIMENSIONAL AND DYNAMIC NATURE OF RESILIENCE

Pioneering research over the past few decades shifted orientation from focusing on stress-related deficits to examining resilience in the face of adversity. Although several disciplines, including neuroscience, psychology, nursing, and medicine, have contributed to the science of resilience, there is to date no universally agreed upon definition (Aburn, Gott, & Hoare, 2016; Fletcher & Sarkar, 2013; Southwick, Bonanno, Masten, Panter-Brick, & Yehuda, 2014).

Investigators looked at resilience using neurobiological and psychological frameworks, and demonstrated the multidimensional and dynamic nature of resilience (Southwick, Litz, Charney, & Friedman, 2011). The multidimensional nature of resilience refers to the research findings that show stressed individuals may be resilient in one aspect of their lives (for example, work), while simultaneously decompensating in another aspect of their lives (for example, intimate relationships). The dynamic nature of resilience refers to uneven expression of resilience throughout one's life. A person may have a resilient response to adversity during one phase of life and then be overcome by challenges presented during another phase of life. Early research indicates resilience is a complex construct that is influenced by social and environmental factors, as well as biological and psychological factors.

For the purpose of this discussion, I refer to the definition of psychological resilience used in *The Sage Encyclopedia of Industrial and Organizational Psychology*,

> Psychological resilience is a person's capacity to maintain a relatively stable equilibrium in the face of adversity. It is the ability of a person to go through difficulties across a continuum of severity . . . and experience relatively minimal abnormal psychological functioning.
>
> (Baran, 2017, p. 1282)

BIOLOGICAL FEATURES OF RESILIENCE

HYPOTHALAMIC-PITUITARY-ADRENAL AXIS

The hypothalamic-pituitary-adrenal axis is the main pathway by which the human body regulates response to stress. When stress is perceived, the hypothalamus secretes corticotropin-releasing hormone (CRH) and arginine-vasopressin. CRH and arginine-vasopressin, in turn, act on the pituitary gland to trigger the release of adrenocorticotropic hormone (ACTH). ACTH then stimulates the adrenal gland to release cortisol and dehydroepiandrosterone (DHEA). Cortisol and DHEA prompt physiologic changes throughout the body, such as arousal, attention, memory formation, and increases in blood glucose and blood pressure, with the goal of supporting the body's ability to cope with the stressor (Harno & White, 2016).

Research shows that resilience may be a product of the efficiency of the cascade of responses along the hypothalamic-pituitary-adrenal axis. Specifically, timely and appropriate activation of the hypothalamic-pituitary-adrenal axis in the presence of a stressor, and deactivation when the stressor is removed, are physiologically adaptive, and promote resilience. A hypoactive or hyperactive response along the hypothalamic-pituitary-adrenal axis leads to disease. Several factors influence the efficiency of the hypothalamic-pituitary-adrenal axis including single nucleotide polymorphisms (SNPs) in genes coding for gamma-aminobutyric acid A receptor, mineralocorticoid receptor, α-adrenoceptor, serotonin transporter, brain-derived neurotrophic factor, and angiotensin-converting enzyme, among others (de Kloet, Derijk, & Meijer, 2007; Derijk, 2009).

MONOAMINE NEUROTRANSMITTERS

Concurrent with activation of the hypothalamic-pituitary-adrenal axis, stress leads to activation of the sympathetic nervous system and inhibition of the parasympathetic nervous system. Consequently, monoamine neurotransmitters, norepinephrine and dopamine are released in response to stress which facilitates encoding emotionally charged memories at the amygdala. Hypersecretion of norepinephrine is associated with anxiety and post-traumatic stress disorder. Another monoamine neurotransmitter, serotonin, has not had its mode of physiologic influence precisely delineated as of yet. That said, it is widely accepted that serotonin metabolites modulate the amygdala and prefrontal cortex to mitigate physiologic responses to stress. Serotonin effects on the body are known to include regulation of anxiety, mood, aggression, and impulse control, and therefore are presumed to contribute to resilience (Krystal & Neumeister, 2009).

Additional agents that appear to modulate the stress response and promote resilience include neuropeptide Y, galanin, testosterone, estrogen, and brain-derived neurotrophic factor. I encourage the reader to pursue elsewhere in-depth study of the biological features of stress and resilience.

BRAIN ARCHITECTURE

There is growing epidemiologic evidence that brain architecture changes over time when children are exposed to toxic stress. Toxic stress is

the excessive or prolonged activation of the physiologic stress response systems in the absence of the buffering protection afforded by stable, responsive relationships. Within the ongoing interplay among assets for health and risks for illness, toxic stress early in life plays a critical role by disrupting brain circuitry and other important regulatory systems in ways that continue to influence physiology, behavior, and health decades later.

(Garner et al., 2012, p. e225)

The following longitudinal study conducted at Washington University School of Medicine provides early evidence of the effects of toxic stress. Researchers enrolled 92 preschoolers, 41 of whom met diagnostic criteria for depression and 51 of whom were healthy (Luby et al., 2012). Investigators objectively measured maternal nurturance and support via structured observations when the children were preschoolers. Several years later, during elementary school, the children received a magnetic resonance imaging (MRI) scan of the brain to assess hippocampal volume. The hippocampus is a region of the brain that is key to memory and stress modulation. The children who had the lowest depression severity and the highest maternal support had the largest hippocampal volume. In contrast, the children with the highest depression severity and the lowest maternal support had the smallest hippocampal volume. This was the first study to provide prospective evidence in humans of the positive effect of early supportive parenting on healthy hippocampal development. Obviously, the study is small and has limitations, but it is an excellent early step in building scientific evidence for the interactions among emotion, behavior, environment, and biology.

EPIGENETICS

Epigenetics is the modification of DNA transcription caused by external factors that leads to changes in gene expression. This often involves chemical modification of histones or DNA by the addition of a methyl group – a process called methylation. Methylation essentially acts to turn the gene off or, to state another way, to inhibit gene expression (Walter & Humpel, 2017). Scholarly inquiry about epigenetic influences on resilience is a relatively new area of study. Research indicates epigenetic changes can effect upregulation and downregulation of stress-response systems with profound and lasting effects (Rozek, Dolinoy, Sartor, & Omenn, 2014). To gain a better understanding of this process, let's look at an epigenetic research study.

Scientists at University of Wisconsin and University of British Columbia collaborated on a prospective study of epigenetic changes (Essex et al., 2013). The researchers interviewed parents of infants and toddlers about their stress levels, including depression, family-expressed anger, parenting stress, and financial stress. Then when the infants and toddlers in the study reached the age of 15 years, researchers measured methylation patterns in cheek-cell DNA. They found that higher stress levels reported by mothers during their child's first year of life correlated with methylation levels on 139 DNA sites in the adolescents. They also discovered 31 sites that correlated with fathers' higher reported stress when their child was 3 to 4 years of age. The study has limitations, including its small sample size of just over 100 teen participants. However, as the first study to use longitudinal data to demonstrate parental adversity during a child's early years leads to measurable changes in the child's epigenome many years later, the researchers have made an important contribution to the literature. We can expect to learn more about the burgeoning field of epigenetics and resilience in the near future.

PSYCHOLOGY OF RESILIENCE

Resilience is commonly seen as a desired outcome, something we aspire to or hope to achieve. Psychosocial scientists, however, conceptualize resilience "as a developmental process or a dynamic capacity rather than as a static outcome or trait" (Yates, Tyrell, & Masten, 2015, p. 774). By conceptualizing resilience as a developmental adaptation to threat, we recognize it as a capacity that can be learned and cultivated, as well as a skill in which we can achieve competence. As a capacity and skill, we must now appreciate that competence in resilience will vary across cultures. For example, a physician assistant working as a solo family medicine provider in a rural community may be challenged by social isolation. Resilience may manifest by joining the softball league, starting a supper club, singing in the community choir, and contributing to an online discussion board with other health professionals. In contrast, a physician assistant working in the emergency department at an urban medical center in a war-torn region may be challenged by the volume of human tragedy that she witnesses on a daily basis. Whereas the rural family medicine physician assistant adapted to his challenges by engaging in social activities, the urban emergency medicine physician assistant will increase her threat by socializing in a war zone. She may need to manifest resilience by engaging in individual, internally oriented activities like silent meditation, yoga, and writing about her clinical experiences and sharing her writing with her colleagues.

POSITIVE PSYCHOLOGY, POSITIVE PERSONAL TRAITS, AND POSITIVE EMOTIONS

Our understanding of the psychology of resilience has accelerated with advancements in the field of positive psychology. Positive psychology, first introduced in 2000 by psychologists Martin Seligman, PhD and Mihaly Csikszentmihalyi, PhD, "is the scientific study of the strengths that enable individuals and communities to thrive" (University of Pennsylvania, 2018a). Positive psychology focuses on positive personal traits and positive emotions. Some examples of positive personal traits include optimism, happiness, self-determination (an individual's perception of autonomy, competence, and interpersonal relatedness), and subjective well-being (an individual's appraisal of his or her life) (Seligman & Csikszentmihalyi, 2000). Positive emotions are emotions that subjectively feel wholesome and do not yield negative affect like depression, despair, or hopelessness. Some examples of positive emotions include joy, contentment, gratitude, serenity, hope, and awe (Cohn, Fredrickson, Brown, Mikels, & Conway, 2009).

Research has shown that positive personal traits and positive emotions are the substrate from which resilience emerges, primarily by supporting effective coping. In other words, when individuals who maintain positive personal traits and regularly experience positive emotions are challenged by a stressful life event, they are likely to engage effective coping strategies that allow them to be resilient and thrive in the presence of adversity (Tugade, Fredrickson, & Barrett, 2004).

There are several psychological strategies that the scientific community accepts as promoting resilience. Although the precise mechanism of action is unknown, the presumption is that activation of the strategies limit the intensity and duration of the stress response (described in the section, Biological Features of Resilience), thereby favorably affecting both psychological state and physiologic response (Turowski, Man, & Cunningham, 2014). Research shows positive psychological states are associated with diminished stress-induced reactivity along the HPA axis and consequently, are posited to promote resilience (Chida & Hamer, 2008; Siegrist et al., 2005). A growing evidence base supports the efficacy of psychological strategies to foster positive psychological states. A recent meta-analysis, which encompassed results from 31,071 participants across 33 studies, found the following psychological strategies to be protective factors for resilience: life satisfaction, optimism, positive affect, self-efficacy, self-esteem, and social support (Lee et al., 2013). Here are the definitions for the six protective factors that the researchers used in the meta-analysis (p. 272):

Life satisfaction: A global assessment of a person's quality of life according to his chosen criteria.

Optimism: The tendency to believe that one will generally experience good outcomes in life.

Positive affect: The extent to which a person feels enthusiastic, active, and alert.

Self-efficacy: People's belief that they have control over their own functioning and over what occurs in the environment.

Self-esteem: Judgments of self-worth, and/or the degree to which people like or dislike themselves.

Social support: The extent to which an individual believes that his/her needs for support, information, and feedback are fulfilled.

While all six protective factors were found to contribute to resilience, self-efficacy and positive affect were the variables most strongly related to high levels of resilience.

TRANSFORMATIVE RESILIENCE

Ama and Stephanie Marston (2018) draw from an interdisciplinary body of evidence to present the idea of transformative resilience. Transformative resilience does not see adversity as a problem to be avoided, but rather as an opportunity for growth. With elements from positive psychology and post-traumatic growth (Calhoun & Tedeschi, 2006), Marston and Marston describe six characteristics of individuals who experience transformative resilience. The characteristics include adaptability, internal locus of control, continual learning, sense of purpose, ability to leverage support, and active engagement. Later in this chapter, we will see how the absence of these characteristics contribute to burnout (see the Burnout in Healthcare section).

SCIENCE OF RESILIENCE SUMMARY

Our brief foray into the science of resilience has shown how complex the concept of resilience is. From a biological viewpoint, the hypothalamic-pituitary-adrenal axis, monoamine neurotransmitters, hormones, and epigenetics, all influence one's ability to manifest resilience. From a psychological perspective, we recognize resilience as a dynamic adaptation to threat, a capacity that can be learned, and a skill in which we can achieve competence within a cultural paradigm. We see positive personal traits and positive emotions that support effective coping in the face of adversity and allow resilience to emerge. Beyond the idea of bouncing back from adversity, transformative resilience posits that adversity can be an opportunity for growth. Finally, we identify protective factors that promote resilience. Later in the chapter, I use the foundational material from the science of resilience to inform our understanding of ways to cultivate resilience among health professionals.

BURNOUT IN HEALTHCARE

Resilience and burnout are on a continuum of health professional responses. Resilience is the prosocial, adaptive response to work conditions; burnout is the dysfunctional response. Between resilience and burnout are the cognitive, emotional, and behavioral highs and lows of professional life. (Note: for discussion of the related constructs, compassion fatigue and vicarious trauma, see chapter 4 Bearing Witness to Suffering, Effects of Witnessing on Health Professionals.) The preponderance of literature refers to burnout as a syndrome with three characteristic features: emotional exhaustion, depersonalization, and loss of meaning in one's work (Maslach, Jackson, & Leiter, 1996). For health professionals, the characteristic features may be discernible as high absenteeism, high workforce turnover, apathy toward work and relationships, treating patients as objects, and having a low sense of personal accomplishment (O'Mahony, 2011; Todaro-Franceschi, 2013).

BURNOUT PREVALENCE DATA

The prevalence of burnout among health professionals is remarkably high. Physicians and nurses are the two professions that have been surveyed most extensively about burnout; prevalence data from health professions other than medicine and nursing are limited.

PHYSICIANS
In the United States, physicians experience burnout at almost twice the rate of individuals who work in other fields. In a large national sample comparing burnout among US physicians and non-physicians, the excessive burnout burden experienced by physicians persists even when controlling for age, gender, and number of hours worked per week (Shanafelt et al., 2015). According to a recent survey conducted by the Mayo Clinic in collaboration with the American Medical Association, approximately 50% of physicians are presently experiencing burnout. When comparing data from surveys conducted in 2011 and 2014, results show a 9% increase in physician burnout over time, even though there was no increase in the median number of hours worked per week by physicians. There was no corresponding increase in burnout among workers in other fields during the same time period. Burnout among physicians is a worldwide phenomenon, with similar prevalence data reported from other countries (Elbarazi, Loney, Yousef, & Elias, 2017; Suner-Soler et al., 2014; Talih, Warakian, Ajaltouni, Shehab, & Tamim, 2016).There is variability in prevalence by specialty with physicians working "at the front lines of care (e.g., emergency medicine, family medicine, general internal medicine, and neurology)" having the highest risk for burnout (Dyrbye et al., 2017, p. 1).

NURSES

Nurses are similarly challenged by professional burnout. Recent studies report a range of nurse burnout rates from a low of approximately 35% (McHugh, Kutney-Lee, Cimiotti, Sloane, & Aiken, 2011) to a high of 86% (Mealer, Burnham, Goode, Rothbaum, & Moss, 2009). As with physicians, prevalence of nurse burnout varies by specialty with critical care and emergency medicine nurses at highest risk. In addition, data indicate that among nurses there are factors beyond specialty that influence burnout, namely excessive workload, inability to participate in decisions, lack of recognition for achievement, paucity of supportive work relationships, and institutional blockades to doing quality, mission-driven, meaningful work that contributes to the larger community (Waddill-Goad, 2016).

OCCUPATIONAL THERAPISTS AND SOCIAL WORKERS

A 2004 study of occupational therapists and social workers in Australia demonstrated no significant differences in burnout between the two professions (Lloyd & King, 2004). Among the 304 occupational therapists and social workers who participated in the study, most experienced high emotional exhaustion scores accompanied by moderate depersonalization scores, and yet they still were able to maintain a high sense of personal accomplishment. A 2003 attempt to collect burnout data from a national sample of occupational therapists in the United States resulted in 37% response rate (Painter, Akroyd, Elliot, & Adams, 2003). The limited sample showed US occupational therapists had a similar burnout pattern to their Australian counterparts – high rates of emotional exhaustion with low rates of depersonalization and the ability to preserve high personal accomplishment in work.

PHYSICAL THERAPISTS

Saudi Arabian researchers conducted a study of burnout prevalence among a national sample of Saudi physical therapists (N = 171; response rate 72.4%) (Al-Imamam & Al-Sobayel, 2014). Results showed moderate rates of all three subscales (emotional exhaustion, depersonalization, and personal accomplishment) and overall burnout rate (combination of high emotional exhaustion, high depersonalization, and low personal accomplishment) of 7.5%.

The first large scale, national study of burnout prevalence among US physical therapists took place in 2015 (Zambo Anderson, Gould-Fogerite, Pratt, & Perlman, 2015). With 1,366 physical therapists responding (21% of those surveyed), results showed 29% of physical therapists experiencing emotional exhaustion, and 13% experiencing burnout (combination of high emotional exhaustion, high depersonalization, and low personal accomplishment scores). In the United States, physical therapist burnout rate is considerably lower than their colleagues in medicine, nursing, social work, and occupational therapy.

PHYSICIAN ASSISTANTS

To date, there does not appear to be a published national sampling of burnout prevalence among physician assistants. A recent study of physician assistants practicing in rural areas of the United States showed 46% scored high on emotional exhaustion, 46% scored high on depersonalization, and yet only 18% scored low on personal accomplishment (Benson et al., 2016). An older study of emergency medicine physician assistants reports 41% of respondents scored high on emotional exhaustion, 34% of respondents scored high on depersonalization, and 66% scored low on personal accomplishment (Bell, Davison, & Sefcik, 2002). These results were comparable to emergency medicine physicians surveyed the same year. No subsequent surveys of emergency medicine physician assistant burnout have been published. In 2014, a research group in Taiwan compared burnout rates across five health professions serving in a regional academic medical center (N = 1,329) (Chou, Li, & Hu, 2014). Their results showed nurses had the highest rate of burnout at 66%, followed by physician assistants at 62%, physicians at 39%, administrative staff at 36%, and medical technicians at 32%.

STUDENTS

Researchers at the Mayo Clinic have published a series of studies looking at burnout among medical students, residents, and early career physicians. Based on national survey data from 4,402 US medical students, they report 44.6% of students scoring high on emotional exhaustion, 37.9% scoring high on depersonalization, and 35.8% scoring low on personal accomplishment (Dyrbye et al., 2014). The overall burnout prevalence rate for US medical students was 49.6%, which is significantly greater than age-matched, college-educated members of the general population (35.7%, $p < .0001$).

Studies show nursing students are less inclined toward burnout than their medical student peers. Researchers conducted a survey study to assess burnout and compassion fatigue among students enrolled in the University of Delaware four-year baccalaureate nursing degree program (N = 436) (Michalec, Diefenbeck, & Mahoney, 2013). Students in all four years of the curriculum reported modest levels of burnout. Of note, the nursing students scored low on the depersonalization scale of the burnout index, meaning it was rare for them to objectify their patients, disengage, and become cynical about patient care. The students also showed high levels of compassion satisfaction. The results from Delaware were corroborated by a study of nursing students in Brazil which investigated the relationship between hardiness and burnout among nursing students (N = 570) at three universities (da Silva et al., 2014). Overall, 24.7% of the sample was experiencing burnout (high emotional exhaustion, high depersonalization, low sense of accomplishment); and 21.9% of the sample had characteristics of a hardy personality. There was a significant ($p = .033$) inverse relationship between burnout frequency and hardiness frequency indicating hardy personality may protect students against burnout.

FALLOUT FROM BURNOUT

When I read the burnout prevalence data for health professionals, I translate the numbers into the faces of my friends, colleagues, and students who have struggled with burnout. And yes, on two occasions in my long clinical career, I experienced burnout. We are dedicated, competent professionals who, for a period of time, had our perception clouded by burnout. The consequences to health professionals, our families and patients, and to society are substantial. Let's first look at some linkages reported in the literature between health professional burnout and untoward consequences, and then discuss interventions to cultivate resilience and prevent burnout.

ALCOHOL USE DISORDER

Alcohol is the most commonly abused chemical substance worldwide. The medical diagnosis, alcohol use disorder, is "a chronic relapsing brain disease characterized by compulsive alcohol use, loss of control over alcohol intake, and a negative emotional state when not using" (National Institute on Alcohol Abuse and Alcoholism, n.d.). Several studies have found associations between health professional burnout and alcohol use disorder. A 2012 study surveyed over 7,000 members of the American College of Surgeons for self-report of alcohol use disorders, clinical depression, the three burnout domains (emotional exhaustion, depersonalization, and low personal achievement), and reporting medical error in the three months prior to the survey (Oreskovich et al., 2012). Results showed 15.4% of surgeons met criteria for moderate or severe alcohol use disorder (13.9% of male surgeons and 25.6% of female surgeons). The surgeons' results are considerably higher than the data reported for the general US population, which shows overall 9.4% of the population meet criteria for all substance misuse, including alcohol. In addition, the gender differential for surgeons with alcohol use disorders is a reversal of what is documented for the general US population, which shows men are more than twice as likely as women are to abuse all substances. Risk for alcohol use disorders among the surgeons increased for those who had burnout, depression, and reported medical error in the three months prior to the survey.

Building on the results from the study of surgeons, the research team applied similar methodology to a survey study of all US physicians (Oreskovich et al., 2015). They surveyed over 7,000 physicians across a variety of specialties to assess chemical substance use (including alcohol), clinical depression, burnout, and reporting medical error in the three months prior to the survey. The results were nearly identical to those reported by the surgeons. The physician survey showed 15.3% of the total sample met criteria for moderate or severe alcohol use disorder. Female physicians were more likely to be afflicted with alcohol use disorders than male physicians (21.4% versus 12.9%). Similar to the surgeons, the physicians demonstrated a strong association between alcohol use disorders and burnout, depression, and reporting a medical error in the three months prior to the survey.

A 2015 study of Danish physicians concurs with several of the findings from the US studies of physicians and surgeons (Pedersen, Sorensen, Bruun, Christensen, & Vedsted, 2016). Similar to the American physicians and surgeons, the Danish physicians met criteria for alcohol use disorders at a much higher rate than the general Dane population (18.8% versus 9%). However, unlike the Americans, Danish male physicians were more likely than female physicians to report chemical substance abuse, including alcohol use disorder. Also similar to the Americans, the Danish physicians demonstrated a strong association between alcohol use disorder and burnout and depression.

Researchers sought to determine the association between alcohol use disorders and distress among US medical students (Jackson, Shanafelt, Hasan, Satele, & Dyrbye, 2016). Using self-report surveys, they elicited information on alcohol use, burnout, depression, suicidal ideation, quality of life, and fatigue. Results showed nearly one-third of the medical student sample met criteria for moderate or severe alcohol use disorder. The medical student rate of alcohol abuse/dependence (32.4%) was more than double that of a sample of US college-educated 22- to 34-year-olds (15.6%), US surgeons (15.4%) (reported earlier), and US physicians (15.3%) (reported earlier). Unlike the studies of physicians and surgeons, the medical students showed no significant gender variability among those meeting criteria for alcohol abuse/dependence (male medical students: 31.8%; female medical students: 32.9%). Similar to the studies of physicians and surgeons, the US medical students showed a strong association between alcohol use disorders and burnout, depression, and low quality of life. Suicidal ideation was higher in the study cohort of medical students (9.4%) than among young adults in the general US population (5.7%); however, the data did not indicate an association between alcohol use disorders and suicidal ideation.

The previous studies indicate physicians, surgeons, and medical students are much more vulnerable to the brain disease, alcohol use disorder, than are other members of society. The association of alcohol use disorder with burnout is a startling reminder that healthcare work conditions are suboptimal for many health professionals. When we consider the increased risk of medical error, as well as the devastation that alcohol dependence invariably bestows on family members and society, it is incumbent on us to find a solution to health professional burnout and alcohol use disorders.

SUICIDAL IDEATION AND SUICIDE

Dutch researchers report a strong correlation between burnout and suicidal ideation (van der Heijden, Dillingh, Bakker, & Prins, 2008). Among the study sample of 2,115 Dutch medical residents, those who met criteria for burnout had a significantly higher prevalence of suicidal thoughts (20.5%) than those who did not meet criteria for burnout (7.6%). Similar results were found among a cohort of Lebanese medical residents (Talih et al., 2016).

Tragically, we have substantial evidence that shows physicians and nurses are significantly more likely to complete suicide than the general population (Alderson, Parent-Rocheleau, & Mishara, 2015; Center et al., 2003; Cheung & Yip, 2016). The striking statistics delimiting the excessive burden of physician and nurse suicide have been apparent for years, yet they remain a closeted secret. Until very recently, the healthcare system has largely ignored or subjugated the heartbreaking loss of life to suicide. We may be at a turning point, however. In 2016, the National Academy of Medicine widely broadcast depression and suicide data, and issued a call for organizational commitment statements to improve clinician well-being. Several august institutions representing physicians, nurses, pharmacists, dentists, health professions educators, academic medical centers, and more responded with action plans and initiatives. Although the link between burnout and suicide has yet to be made, some researchers have found an association between health professional burnout and hopelessness – which is considered a risk factor for suicide (Pomili et al., 2006).

MEDICAL ERROR

Research demonstrates an association between burnout and healthcare quality and safety. Surgeons who are experiencing burnout are more likely to report a major medical error in the *previous* three months than those who are not experiencing burnout (Shanafelt et al., 2010). Likewise, a prospective study of internal medicine residents noted individuals who had high levels of burnout had increased odds of reporting a medical error in the *subsequent* three months. The relationship between burnout and medical error is most likely bidirectional as evidenced by a correlation between self-perceived medical errors and worsening burnout (West et al., 2006; West, Tan, Habermann, Sloan, & Shanafelt, 2009). Another study shows a strong, independent correlation between burnout levels of hospital nurses and patients' urinary tract infections and surgical site infections (Cimiotti, Aiken, Sloane, & Wu, 2012). The authors hypothesize "the cognitive detachment associated with high levels of burnout may result in inadequate hand hygiene practices and lapses in other infection control procedures among registered nurses" (p. 488).

For more than a decade, with healthcare reform at the fore of the national conversation in the United States, the stated "Triple Aim" of the US healthcare system has been to simultaneously pursue three performance indicators: improve the health of populations, increase patient satisfaction via improved quality and safety, and reduce costs (Berwick, Nolan, & Whittington, 2008). Recognizing health professional burnout as a deterrent to achieving the Triple Aim, Thomas Bodeneheimer MD and Christine Sinsky, MD (2014) propose adding a fourth aim. They specify health professional well-being as a prerequisite to quality, safe care that improves the health of populations, and thereby advocate for the Quadruple Aim, which adds improving the work life of health professionals. Sikka, Morath, and Leape (2015) have published a position paper that also calls for an expansion to the Quadruple Aim. The authors state, "The key is the fourth aim: creating the conditions for the healthcare workforce to find joy and meaning in their work and in doing so, improving the experience of providing care" (p. 609).

CONSEQUENCES OF BURNOUT: SUMMARY

We have unambiguous evidence about the consequences of burnout to health professionals, families, patients, and society. The evidence demands the question: Are burnout and loss of life to suicide a reflection of a healthcare system in crisis? It is easy for me to grow sad and fearful of a healthcare system that perpetuates work conditions that are conducive to burnout, and neglects to institute a concerted and coordinated effort to prevent health professional suicide. However, I derive encouragement from the idea that increased awareness leads to a groundswell of support for preventive measures. I hope this chapter contributes to awareness of the burden carried by many health professionals and acts as a call to intervene. As health professionals, we must take care of ourselves and each other. It is literally a matter of life and death.

Let's look at some efficacious interventions that can be helpful to individual health professionals, and may eventually change the healthcare system.

INTERVENTIONS TO CULTIVATE RESILIENCE

RESILIENCE COMPETENCIES

Led by efforts at the Penn Resilience Program, University of Pennsylvania Positive Psychology Center, there is a robust research base to support implementation of resilience programming in a variety of settings. Generally speaking, the aim of the programming is to identify and enhance a resilience skill set that promotes resilience competencies. The resilience competencies are:

1 develop self-awareness of one's thoughts, emotions, and behaviors;
2 engage in self-regulation of impulsive thoughts and behaviors, as well as the willingness and ability to express emotions;
3 have reality-based optimism, noticing the good in oneself and others and challenging counterproductive beliefs;
4 developmental agility – as in being able to think flexibly and to take another's perspective;
5 rely on character strengths – which means to know one's strengths and be able to use them to surmount challenges;
6 build connections and strong relationships through communication, empathy, and the ability to ask for help. (University of Pennsylvania, 2018b)

RESILIENCE FACTORS

Yale School of Medicine professor, Stephen Southwick, MD and Dean of Icahn School of Medicine at Mount Sinai, Dennis Charney, MD have distilled years of work with people who have experienced trauma to learn key approaches to cultivating resilience. In their text, *Resilience: The Science of Mastering Life's Greatest Challenges,* they describe interviews they conducted with prisoners of war, members of the US Army Special Forces, and individuals who had experienced congenital disorders, childhood sexual abuse, death of parents in childhood, abduction and rape, loss of limb, and cancer. Southwick and Charney (2012, p. 11) analyzed the interviews to identify ten coping mechanisms, which they refer to as resilience factors.

all of the individuals we interviewed confronted their fears, maintained an optimistic but realistic outlook, sought and accepted social support, and imitated sturdy role models. Most also relied upon their own inner moral compass, turned to religious or spiritual practices, and found a way to accept that which they could not change. Many attended to their health and well-being, and trained intensively to stay physically fit, mentally sharp, and emotionally strong. And most were active problem solvers who looked for meaning and opportunity in the midst of adversity and sometime even found humor in the darkness. Finally, all of the resilient people we interviewed accepted, to an impressive degree, responsibility for their own emotional well-being, and many used their traumatic experiences as a platform for personal growth.

If you compare Southwick and Charney's resilience factors to the Penn Resilience Program resilience competencies (described earlier), you will notice considerable concurrence. Southwick and Charney add three more factors: humor, active engagement in problem-solving, and imitating role models. Over the course of my clinical career, I have met many patients who have been role models of resilience. These are people who have embraced the whole messy mystery of life, illness, disability, and death with awareness, attention, curiosity, and authenticity. At the conclusion of this chapter, I provide a learner activity that centers upon patients who can be role models of resilience for us.

RESILIENCE CULTIVATION PROGRAMS

In this section, we look in detail at a few of the successful resilience cultivation programs that target health professionals and health professional students specifically, and help us maintain personal well-being, empathy for our patients and colleagues, and meaning in our work. Notice that the six resilience competencies listed earlier and the resilience cultivation programs described later intervene at the level of the individual. In effect they aim to teach individuals how to survive in a flawed system – in my estimation, that is solving the wrong problem. The truly humane approach to health professional burnout and its consequences is to intervene at the system level (Shanafelt, Dyrbye, & West, 2017; Shanafelt & Noseworthy, 2017). We need a healthcare system that respects health professionals and gives us time and space to create meaningful relationships with patients and colleagues, understands our human limitations and safeguards against our inevitable mistakes, and grants us permission to care for ourselves and our families. I consider the individual-level resilience interventions described later in this chapter to be stopgap measures that will perhaps ease the life-threatening misery experienced by many health professionals while we simultaneously overhaul the system in which we try to work.

DISCUSSION GROUP, REFLECTION, NARRATIVE STUDY, AND MINDFULNESS MEDITATION

The Mayo Clinic has conducted a series of small studies to reduce burnout and promote resilience. In one randomized controlled trial, physicians in the department of medicine (N = 74) were randomly assigned to a control or intervention arm for the nine month study period (West et al., 2014). Participants in the control arm received one hour of paid protected time biweekly that they could use however they chose. Participants in the intervention arm attended biweekly one hour facilitated discussion groups. The curriculum for the discussion groups encompassed "meaning in work, personal and professional balance, medical mistakes, community, caring for patients, and other topics relevant to practicing physicians" (p. 528). The groups provided the opportunity for reflection, writing, sharing, and the practice of mindfulness. Outcomes were measured at baseline, every three months during the intervention period, and three months and twelve months post-intervention period. Self-report surveys were used to assess meaning in work (including empowerment and engagement), quality of life, physical and psychological well-being, depression, perceived stress, and burnout. Results showed participants in the small group discussion had significantly improved meaning in work, including engagement and empowerment, during the intervention period and sustained over time as compared to the control participants who were afforded an hour of free time. Similarly, the small group intervention participants had improvement in their burnout scores compared to the control participants, which were also maintained one year post-intervention. Of note, the intervention group did not experience a change in their perceived stress, quality of life, or depression scores, indicating their work conditions remained challenging during this time period.

MINDFULNESS MEDITATION, NARRATIVE MEDICINE, AND APPRECIATIVE INQUIRY

The University of Rochester Medical Center conducted a mindful communication intervention for primary care physicians (N = 70), with the aim to improve physician well-being, psychological distress, burnout, and capacity to relate to patients (Krasner et al., 2009). The intervention consisted of eight weekly 2.5 hour facilitated discussions and one full day silent retreat, followed by monthly meetings for 10 months. The curriculum was framed by didactic sessions on topics such as "awareness of thoughts and feelings, perceptual biases and filters, dealing with pleasant and unpleasant events, managing conflict, preventing burnout, reflecting on meaningful experiences in practice, setting boundaries, examining attraction to patients, exploring self-care, being with suffering, and examining end-of-life care" (p. 1285). The experiential activities, selected to aid participants in developing self-awareness, included mindfulness meditation practice, narrative medicine methods of close reading, writing, and sharing, and appreciative inquiry techniques. Outcome measures, completed at baseline, 2 months, 12 months, and 15 months, included self-report surveys of burnout, mood, emotional stability, mindfulness, and patient-centered attitudes (empathy and psychosocial orientation). Results showed participants experienced diminished burnout, improved mood, and positive changes in patient-centered attitudes (empathy and psychosocial orientation). Most of the improvements were maintained beyond the intervention period.

In follow-up to the intervention study, the researchers at University of Rochester Medical Center conducted qualitative interviews with a subset of the participants (N = 20) to determine the components of the intervention the physicians perceived as most helpful to their well-being and clinical practice (Beckman et al., 2012). The qualitative assessment revealed three themes, "1) professional isolation from colleagues and a desire to share their experiences, 2) acquiring skills of attentiveness, listening, honesty, and presence, and 3) taking time for professional and personal development" (p. 816). Participants explicitly described the joy, pleasure, and support they derived from the group intervention. They also talked about the positive impact of learning, practicing, and applying mindfulness skills, including increased capacity to listen and be attentive, open, self-aware, and empathetic with patients, colleagues, and their families. They also said the narrative medicine activities helped them develop proficiency in being able to share medical errors, grief, and sorrow with colleagues, and that many of the encounters with members of their group were "profoundly transformative" (p. 817). Participants were deeply appreciative of the dedicated time to care for themselves and refuel for their patients and families.

Researchers in Spain used the University of Rochester Medical Center mindful communication intervention protocol (described earlier) for a randomized controlled trial of primary care physicians and nurses (N = 68) who worked in the Spanish public health system (Asuero et al., 2014). Similar to the results attained by the Rochester researchers, the Spanish intervention cohort showed significant improvement in mood and mindfulness scores, and moderate improvement in burnout and empathy scores, while the control group demonstrated no change over the study period.

ONLINE MIND-BODY SKILLS TRAINING (RELAXATION RESPONSE, MINDFULNESS, AUTOGENIC TRAINING, POSITIVE AFFECT MEDITATION)

A large academic medical center in Midwestern United States offered free, elective, online mind-body skills training for health professionals at their institution (Kemper & Khirallah, 2015). The aim of the study was to assess the appeal of online training and the effects of the training on health professional stress, resilience, and burnout. The study sample (N = 513) included dietitians, nurses, physicians, social workers, clinical trainees, and health researchers. "The training included up to 12 one-hour modules, three for each of four types of mind – body skills: (a) focused attention meditation (relaxation response), (b) mindfulness, (c) guided imagery and hypnosis (including autogenic training), and (d) positive affect – generating meditation (such as gratitude and loving-kindness)" (p. 248). Participants were allowed to take any combination of modules, in any order they chose. Outcome measures included self-report surveys, completed at baseline and at the end of the training, for burnout, stress, mindful attention, resilience, empathy, and perspective taking. At baseline, participants reported high levels of perceived stress and burnout, and had below average scores for resilience – indicating the training had appeal for health professionals who were likely in need of an intervention. At the conclusion of the training, scores improved significantly for perceived stress, resilience, mindful attention, empathy, and perspective-taking scores.

MINDFULNESS-BASED STRESS REDUCTION

Researchers in Portugal studied the effect of a six-week mindfulness-based stress reduction program on burnout, compassion fatigue, mood, mindfulness, and self-compassion among oncology nurses (N = 93) (Duarte & Pinto-Gouveia, 2016). Participants were assigned to either the intervention group or waitlist control group. The intervention curriculum covered mindfulness practices focused on the breath, body, difficult emotions, and thoughts, as well as loving-kindness meditation, and mindful communication. Participants were given a CD with guided meditations and were instructed to practice daily at home. Self-report outcome measures, completed at baseline and post-intervention, showed significant decreases in burnout, perceived stress, and compassion fatigue among the intervention group as compared to the control group.

RESILIENCE INTERVENTION RESEARCH: SUMMARY

As you can see from the intervention research described in this chapter, researchers from various institutions have chosen to include mindfulness practices and narrative study (in different iterations and combinations) as core intervention content to address burnout and cultivate resilience. Professor Johanna Shapiro, from University of California, Irvine School of Medicine, writes about medical students' distress and emotional dysregulation when they encounter their own and their patients' intense feelings in the clinical setting. Professor Shapiro describes ways medical students can learn to work skillfully with emotions and build resilience. Similar to the Penn Resilience Program and Southwick and Charney's resilience factors (described earlier), Dr. Shapiro calls for emotional awareness, emotion regulation, and interpersonal connection to achieve clinical empathy. She points to mindfulness meditation and narrative medicine as two effective ways of cultivating resilience within medical education. Dr. Shapiro (2011, p. 330) writes,

> The relevant premise behind such humanities-based teaching strategies is that, by engaging with and encouraging reflection on the emotions, the humanities create familiarity with emotional landscapes as well as an awareness of how the interplay of emotions in clinical settings affects both patient and physician.

Research on individual resilience interventions is promising, though still in its infancy. Generally speaking, the studies to date have been small and suffer from high attrition. The studies often lack appropriate multivariate statistical analysis, fail to control for potential confounders, and neglect to identify interaction effects among variables (Dyrbye et al., 2017). Two recent meta-analyses show modest effect from individual interventions to prevent burnout and/or promote resilience among physicians (Panagioti et al., 2017; West, Dyrbye, Erwin, & Shanafelt, 2016). The meta-analytic results further support the premise that individual interventions are insufficient to address health professional burnout. We must pursue system-level interventions if we are to adequately curtail the egregious consequences of burnout on health professionals, patients, and society.

CLOSING

In this chapter, we looked at the biological and psychological features of resilience. We compared resilience and burnout, reviewed the prevalence data on health professional burnout, and examined the profound burden carried by health professionals, families, and society from the consequences of burnout. We looked at resilience competencies and resilience factors as protection against burnout, and then reviewed some effective individual resilience intervention studies. We highlighted the need for system-level interventions to address the work conditions that hinder meaningful, safe healthcare.

I close this chapter with learning objectives and activities that provide the reader with the opportunity to explore resilience in our patients. Patients who find creative ways to adapt and grow in the presence of life-altering disease can be our positive role models for resilience.

ACTIVITIES

LEARNING OBJECTIVES

Learners will

1 explore the concept of resilience in the context of healthcare;
2 recognize the attitudes and behaviors that cultivate resilience;
3 reflect on their personal experience of resilience.

PHOTOGALLERY AND DISCUSSION

First, view photographs from *The Scar Project* of young women who have been scarred by breast cancer. *The Scar Project* is an initiative to heighten awareness about breast cancer. The project's tagline is: "Breast Cancer is Not a Pink Ribbon." The project was started by a professional fashion photographer, David Jay, whose close friend was diagnosed with breast cancer. His mission is to reveal raw truths about cancer, demonstrate how much the women have at stake, and show their humanity. Women have traveled to New York from all over to be part of the project. A traveling exhibit of the photographs has been displayed in museums throughout the world. There is also a documentary film (Zagarella & Zagarella, 2011) and book (Jay, 2011) about *The Scar Project* and the women who participated.

The photos show the women in partial nudity – and they are uncompromisingly honest. It can be difficult to look. You decide if you need to look away. If you are able to look – ask yourself, what do I see? If you have to look away, ask yourself why?

The photogallery is available at www.thescarproject.org/gallery/

SMALL GROUP DISCUSSION

Learners are invited to discuss their experience with the photogallery. Whenever possible, learners should refer to specific photographs. In particular, learners should aim to comment on the qualities of resilience.

NOTE: **Appendix A** has general guidelines for facilitating a health humanities seminar. **Appendix B** has instruction and discussion prompts specific to this activity for faculty facilitators to use if your learners are not able to initiate a robust discussion.

WRITING AND SHARING

The second activity is for the learner to write to a prompt that directly links the chapter content and the photogallery. Here is a suggested writing prompt:

Write about one of your scars. Feel free to write fiction.

Faculty facilitators can invite the learners to share what they have written with the group. Learners should never be required to share their writings.

REFERENCE LIST

Aburn, G., Gott, M., & Hoare, K. (2016). What is resilience? An integrative review of the empirical literature. *Journal of Advanced Nursing, 72*(5), 980–1000.

Al-Imamam, D. M., & Al-Sobayel, H. A. (2014). The prevalence and severity of burnout among physiotherapists in an Arabian setting and the influence of organizational factors: An observational study. *Journal of Physical Therapy Science, 26*, 1193–1198.

Alderson, M., Parent-Rocheleau, X., & Mishara, B. (2015). Critical review on suicide among nurses: What about work-related factors? *Crisis, 36*(2), 91–101.

Asuero, A. M., Queralto, J. M., Pujol-Ribera, E., Berenguera, A., Rodriguez-Blanco, T., & Epstein, R. M. (2014). Effectiveness of a mindfulness education program in primary health care professionals: A pragmatic controlled trial. *Journal of Continuing Education in the Health Professions, 34*(1), 4–12.

Baran, B. E. (2017). Psychological resilience. In S. E. Rogelberg (Ed.), *The Sage encyclopedia of industrial and organizational psychology* (2nd ed.). Thousand Oaks, CA: Sage.

Beckman, H. B., Wendland, M., Mooney, C., Krasner, M. S., Quill, T. E., Suchman, A. L., & Epstein, R. M. (2012). The impact of a program in mindful communication on primary care physicians. *Academic Medicine, 87*(6), 815–819.

Bell, R. B., Davison, M., & Sefcik, D. (2002). A first survey measuring burnout in emergency medicine physician assistants. *JAAPA, 15*(3), 40–55.

Benson, M. A., Peterson, T., Salazar, L., Morris, W., Hall, R., Howlett, B., & Phelps, P. (2016). Burnout in rural physician assistants: An initial study. *Journal of Physician Assistant Education, 27*(2), 81–83.

Berwick, D. M., Nolan, T. W., & Whittington, J. (2008). The Triple Aim: Care, health, and cost. *Health Affairs, 27*(3), 759–769.

Bodenheimer, T., & Sinsky, C. (2014). From Triple to Quadruple Aim: Care of the patient requires care of the provider. *Annals of Family Medicine, 12*, 573–576.

Calhoun, L. G., & Tedeschi, R. G. (Eds.). (2006). *The handbook of posttraumatic growth: Research and practice.* Mahwah, NJ: Lawrence Erlbaum Associates.

Center, C., Davis, M., Detre, T., Ford, D. E., Hansbrough, W., Hendin, H., . . . Silverman, M. M. (2003). Confronting depression and suicide in physicians: A consensus statement. *JAMA, 289*, 3161–3166.

Cheung, T., & Yip, P. S. F. (2016). Self-harm in nurses: Prevalence and correlates. *Journal of Advanced Nursing, 72*(9), 2124–2137.

Chida, Y., & Hamer, M. (2008). Chronic psychosocial factors and acute physiological responses to laboratory-induced stress in healthy populations: A quantitative review of 30 years of investigations. *Psychological Bulletin, 134*, 829–885.

Chou, L., Li, C., & Hu, S. C. (2014). Job stress and burnout in hospital employees: Comparisons of different medical professions in a regional hospital in Taiwan. *BMJ Open, 4*, e004185. doi:10.1136/ bmjopen-2013-004185

Cimiotti, J. P., Aiken, L. H., Sloane, D. M., & Wu, E. S. (2012). Nurse staffing, burnout, and health care-associated infection. *American Journal of Infection Control, 40*, 486–490.

Cohn, M. A., Fredrickson, B. L., Brown, S. L., Mikels, J. A., & Conway, A. M. (2009). Happiness unpacked: Positive emotions increase life satisfaction by building resilience. *Emotion, 9*(3), 361–368.

da Silva, R. M., Goulart, C. T., Dias Lopes, L. F., Serrano, P. M., Siqueira Costa, A. L., & de Azevedo Guido, L. (2014). Hardy personality and burnout syndrome among nursing students in three Brazilian universities – An analytic study. *Biomedical Central Nursing, 13*(9). doi:10.1186/1472-6955-13-9

de Kloet, E. R., Derijk, R. H., & Meijer, O. C. (2007). Therapy insight: Is there an imbalanced response of mineralocorticoid and glucocorticoid receptors in depression? *Nature Clinical and Practical Endocrinology and Metabolism, 3*, 168–179.

Derijk, R. H. (2009). Single nucleotide polymorphisms related to HPA axis reactivity. *Neuroimmunomodulation, 6*, 340–352.

Duarte, J., & Pinto-Gouveia, J. (2016). Effectiveness of a mindfulness-based intervention on oncology nurses' burnout and compassion fatigue symptoms: A non-randomized study. *International Journal of Nursing Studies, 64*, 98–107.

Dyrbye, L. N., Shanafelt, T. D., Sinsky, C. A., Cipriano, P. F., Bhatt, J., Ommaya, A., West, C. P., & Meyers, D. (2017). Burnout among health care professionals: A call to explore and address this underrecognized threat to safe, high-quality care. In *NAM Perspectives*. Washington, DC: National Academy of Medicine. Retrieved from https://nam.edu/wp-content/uploads/2017/07/Burnout-Among-Health-Care-Professionals-A-Call-to-Explore-and-Address-This-Underrecognized-Threat.pdf

Dyrbye, L. N., West, C. P., Satele, D., Boone, S., Tan, L., Sloan, J., & Shanafelt, T. D. (2014). Burnout among US medical students, residents, and early career physicians relative to the general US population. *Academic Medicine, 89*, 443–451.

Elbarazi, I., Loney, T., Yousef, S., & Elias, A. (2017). Prevalence of and factors associated with burnout among health care professionals in Arab countries: A systematic review. *BMC Health Services Research, 17*, 491. doi:10.1186/s12913-017-2319-8

Essex, M. J., Boyce, W. T., Hertzman, C., Lam, L. L., Armstrong, J. M., Neumann, S. M. A., & Kobor, M. S. (2013). Epigenetic vestiges of early developmental adversity: Childhood stress exposure and DNA methylation in adolescence. *Child Development, 84*(1), 58–75.

Fletcher, D., & Sarkar, M. (2013). Psychological resilience: A review and critique of definitions, concepts, and theory. *European Psychologist, 18*(1), 12–23.

Garner, A. S., Shonkoff, J. P., Siegel, B. S., Dobbins, M. I., Earls, M. F., McGuinn, L., . . . Wood, D. L. (2012). Early childhood adversity, toxic stress, and the role of the pediatrician: Translating developmental science into lifelong health. *Pediatrics, 129*(1), e224–e231. doi:10.1542/peds.2011-2662

Harno, E., & White, A. (2016). Adrenocorticotropic hormone. In J. L. Jameson & L. J. de Groot (Eds.), *Endocrinology: Adult and pediatric, volume 1* (7th ed., pp. 129–146). Philadelphia, PA: Elsevier Saunders.

Jackson, E. R., Shanafelt, T. D., Hasan, O., Satele, D. V., & Dyrbye, L. N. (2016). Burnout and alcohol abuse/dependence among US medical students. *Academic Medicine, 91*, 1251–1256.

Jay, D. (2011). *The Scar Project: Breast cancer is not a pink ribbon.* New York: The Scar Project.

Kemper, K. J., & Khirallah, M. (2015). Acute effects of online mind-body skills training on resilience, mindfulness, and empathy. *Journal of Evidence-Based Complementary and Alternative Medicine, 20*(4), 247–253.

Krasner, M. S., Epstein, R. M., Beckman, H., Suchman, A. L., Chapman, B., Mooney, C. J., & Quill, T. E. (2009). Association of an educational program in mindful communication with burnout, empathy, and attitudes among primary care physicians. *JAMA, 302*(12), 1284–1293.

Krystal, J. H., & Neumeister, A. (2009). Noradrenergic and serotonergic mechanisms in the neurobiology of posttraumatic stress disorder and resilience. *Brain Research, 1293*, 13–23.

Lee, J. H., Nam, S. K., Kim, A. R., Kim, B., Lee, M. Y., & Lee, S. M. (2013). Resilience: A meta-analytic approach. *Journal of Counseling and Development, 91*(3), 269–279.

Lloyd, C., & King, R. (2004). A survey of burnout among Australian mental health occupational therapists and social workers. *Social Psychiatry and Psychiatric Epidemiology, 39*, 752–757.

Luby, J. L., Barch, D. M., Belden, A., Gaffrey, M. S., Tillman, R., Babb, C., Nishino, T., Suzuki, H., & Botteron, K. N. (2012). Maternal support in early childhood predicts larger hippocampal volumes at school age. *Proceedings of the National Academy of Sciences of the USA, 109*(8), 2854–2859.

Marston, A., & Marston, S. (2018). *Type R: Transformative resilience for thriving in a turbulent world.* New York: Public Affairs Books.

Maslach, C., Jackson, S. E., & Leiter, M. P. (1996). *Maslach Burnout inventory manual* (3rd ed.). Palo Alto, CA: Consulting Psychologists.

McHugh, M. D., Kutney-Lee, A., Cimiotti, J. P., Sloane, D. M., & Aiken, L. H. (2011). Nurses' widespread job dissatisfaction, burnout, and frustration with health benefits signal problems for patient care. *Health Affairs, 30*, 202–210.

Mealer, M., Burnham, E. L., Goode, C. J., Rothbaum, B., & Moss, M. (2009). The prevalence and impact of post traumatic stress disorder and burnout syndrome in nurses. *Depression and Anxiety, 26*, 1118–1126.

Michalec, B., Diefenbeck, C., & Mahoney, M. (2013). The calm before the storm? Burnout and compassion fatigue among undergraduate nursing students. *Nurse Education Today, 33*, 314–320.

National Academy of Medicine. (2016). *Action collaborative on clinician well-being and resilience.* Author. Retrieved from https://nam.edu/initiatives/clinician-resilience-and-well-being/commitment-statements-clinician-well-being/

National Institute on Alcohol Abuse and Alcoholism. (n.d.). *Alcohol use disorder.* Author. Retrieved from www.niaaa.nih.gov/alcohol-health/overview-alcohol-consumption/alcohol-use-disorders

O'Mahony, N. (2011). Nurse burnout and the working environment. *Emergency Nurse, 19*(5), 30–37.

Oreskovich, M. R., Kaups, K. L., Balch, C. M., Hanks, J. B., Satele, D., Sloan, J., . . . Shanafelt, T. D. (2012). Prevalence of alcohol use disorders among American surgeons. *Archives of Surgery, 147*(2), 168–174.

Oreskovich, M. R., Shanafelt, T., Dyrbye, L. N., Tan, L., Sotile, W., Satele, D., . . . Boone, S. (2015). The prevalence of substance use disorders in American physicians. *The American Journal on Addictions, 24*, 30–38.

Painter, J., Akroyd, D., Elliot, S., & Adams, R. D. (2003). Burnout among occupational therapists. *Occupational Therapy in Health Care, 17*, 63–78.

Panagioti, M., Panagopoulou, E., Bower, P., Lewith, G., Kontopantelis, E., Chew-Graham, C., Dawson, S., Marwijk, H., Geraghty, K., & Esmail, A. (2017). Controlled interventions to reduce burnout in physicians: A systematic review and meta-analysis. *JAMA Internal Medicine, 177*(2), 195–205.

Pedersen, A. F., Sorensen, J. K., Bruun, N. H., Christensen, B., & Vedsted, P. (2016). Risky alcohol use in Danish physicians: Associated with alexithymia and burnout? *Drug and Alcohol Dependence, 160*, 119–126.

Pomili, M., Rinaldi, G., Lester, D., Girardi, P., Ruberto, A., & Tatarelli, R. (2006). Hopelessness and suicide risk emerge in psychiatric nurses suffering from burnout and using specific defense mechanisms. *Archives of Psychiatric Nursing, 20*(3), 135–143.

Rozek, L. S., Dolinoy, D. C., Sartor, M. A., & Omenn, G. S. (2014). Epigenetics: Relevance and implications for public health. *Annual Review of Public Health, 35*, 105–122.

Seligman, M., & Csikszentmihalyi, M. (2000). Positive psychology: An introduction. *American Psychologist, 55*(1), 5–14.

Shanafelt, T. D., Balch, C. M., Bechamps, G., Russell, T., Dyrbye, L., Satele, D., . . . Freischlag, J. (2010). Burnout and medical errors among American surgeons. *Annals of Surgery, 251*, 995–1000.

Shanafelt, T. D., Dyrbye, L. N., & West, C. P. (2017). Addressing physician burnout: The way forward. *JAMA, 317*(9), 901–902.

Shanafelt, T. D., Hasan, O., Dyrbye, L. N., Sinsky, C., Satele, D., Sloan, J., & West, C. P. (2015). Changes in burnout and satisfaction with work-life balance in physicians and the general US working population between 2011 and 2014. *Mayo Clinic Proceedings, 90*(12), 1600–1613.

Shanafelt, T. D., & Noseworthy, J. H. (2017). Executive leadership and physician well-being: Nine organizational strategies to promote engagement and reduce burnout. *Mayo Clinic Proceedings, 92*(1), 129–146.

Shapiro, J. (2011). Does medical education promote professional alexithymia? A call for attending to the emotions of patients and self in medical training. *Academic Medicine, 86*(3), 326–332.

Siegrist, J., Menrath, I., Stocker, T., Klein, M., Kellermann, T., Shah, N. J., Zilles, K., & Schneider, F. (2005). Differential brain activation according to chronic social reward frustration. *NeuroReport, 16*(17), 1899–1903.

Sikka, R., Morath, J. M., & Leape, L. (2015). The Quadruple Aim: Care, health, cost and meaning in work. *BMJ Quality & Safety, 24,* 608–610.

Southwick, S. M., Bonanno, G. A., Masten, A. S., Panter-Brick, C., & Yehuda, R. (2014). Resilience definitions, theory, and challenges: Interdisciplinary perspectives. *European Journal of Psychotraumatology, 5,* 1, 25338. doi:10.3402/ejpt.v5.25338

Southwick, S. M., & Charney, D. (2012). *Resilience: The science of mastering life's greatest challenges.* New York: Cambridge University Press.

Southwick, S. M., Litz, B. T., Charney, D., & Friedman, M. J. (Eds.). (2011). *Resilience and mental health: Challenges across the lifespan.* New York: Cambridge University Press.

Suner-Soler, R., Grau-Martin, A., Flichtentrei, D., Prats, M., Braga, F., Font-Mayolas, S., & Gras, M. E. (2014). The consequences of burnout syndrome among healthcare professionals in Spain and Spanish speaking Latin American countries. *Burnout Research, 1,* 82–89.

Talih, F., Warakian, R., Ajaltouni, J., Shehab, A. A. S., & Tamim, H. (2016). Correlates of depression and burnout among residents in a Lebanese academic medical center: A cross-sectional study. *Academic Psychiatry, 40,* 38–45.

Todaro-Franceschi, V. (2013). *Compassion fatigue and burnout in nursing: Enhancing professional quality of life.* New York: Springer.

Tugade, M. M., Fredrickson, B. L., & Barrett, L. F. (2004). Psychological resilience and positive emotional granularity: Examining the benefits of positive emotions on coping and health. *Journal of Personality, 72*(6), 1161–1190.

Turowski, T. K., Man, V. Y., & Cunningham, W. A. (2014). Positive emotion and the brain: The neuroscience of happiness. In J. Gruber & J. T. Moskowitz (Eds.), *Positive emotion: Integrating the light sides and dark sides* (pp. 95–115). New York: Oxford University Press.

University of Pennsylvania. (2018a). *Positive psychology center.* The Trustees of the University of Pennsylvania. Retrieved from https://ppc.sas.upenn.edu/

University of Pennsylvania. (2018b). *Resilience skill set.* The Trustees of the University of Pennsylvania. Retrieved from https://ppc.sas.upenn.edu/resilience-programs/resilience-skill-set

van der Heijden, F., Dillingh, G., Bakker, A., & Prins, J. (2008). Suicidal thoughts among medical residents with burnout. *Archives of Suicide Research, 12,* 344–346.

Waddill-Goad, S. (2016). *Nurse burnout: Combating stress in nursing.* Indianapolis, IN: Sigma Theta Tau International.

Walter, J., & Humpel, A. (2017). Introduction to epigenetics. In R. Heil, S. Seitz, H. Konig, & J. Robienski (Eds.), *Epigenetics: Ethical, legal, and social aspects* (pp. 11–30). Wiesbaden, DE: Springer VS.

West, C. P., Dyrbye, L. N., Erwin, P. J., & Shanafelt, T. D. (2016). Interventions to prevent and reduce physician burnout: A systematic review and meta-analysis. *Lancet, 388,* 2272–2281.

West, C. P., Dyrbye, L. N., Rabatin, J. T., Call, T. G., Davidson, J. H., Multari, A., . . . Shanafelt, T. D. (2014). Intervention to promote physician well-being, job satisfaction, and professionalism. *JAMA Internal Medicine, 174*(4), 527–533.

West, C. P., Huschka, M., Novotny, P., Sloan, J. A., Kolars, C., Habermann, T. M., & Shanafelt, T. D. (2006). Association of perceived medical errors with resident distress and empathy: A prospective longitudinal study. *JAMA, 296*(9), 1071–1078.

West, C. P., Tan, A. D., Habermann, T. M., Sloan, J. A., & Shanafelt, T. D. (2009). Association of resident fatigue and distress with perceived medical errors. *JAMA, 302,* 1294–1300.

Yates, T. M., Tyrell, F. A., & Masten, A. S. (2015). Resilience theory and the practice of positive psychology from individuals to societies. In S. Joseph (Ed.), *Positive psychology in practice: Promoting human flourishing in work, health, education, and everyday life* (2nd ed.) (doi:10.1002/9781118996874.ch44). Hoboken, NJ: John Wiley & Sons.

Zagarella, P. (producer), & Zagarella, P. (director). (2011). *Baring it all (They came from all over).* Lost in Vision Entertainment.

Zambo Anderson, E., Gould-Fogerite, S., Pratt, C., & Perlman, A. (2015). Identifying stress and burnout in physical therapists. *Physiotherapy, 101*(supplement 1), e1712–e1713. doi:10.1016/j.physio.2015.03.126

6 RECOGNIZING OUR INTERDEPENDENCE

> INTEGRATION NOTE
> ....
> This chapter integrates with curricula on health professional–patient communication, health professional well-being, and professionalism. The learner activity at the end of the chapter complements instruction related to cancer care.

INTRODUCTION

By virtue of our professional ethic and responsibilities, and the very nature of healthcare, societal expectation is that the attitude and actions of the health professional will affect the patient – ideally with a positive outcome. The patient depends on the health professional to be knowledgeable and skillful, and trusts the health professional to bring honorable intentions to the relationship. The expectation is *not* interdependence, but rather unidirectional dependence. Interdependence refers to a relationship in which the attitude and actions of each person depend on the other person. Interdependence is bidirectional and includes a mutuality of behaviors and outcomes. For interdependence to occur in the clinical setting, the health professional and patient need to influence the relationship mutually. Although the health professional's effect on patient outcomes, both positive and negative, are expected, obvious, and reasonably well researched, the patient's effect on health professional outcomes has received far less attention to date.

Research has focused on characterizing and deconstructing the complexities of the health professional–patient relationship, with most attention levied on physicians and nurses at the exclusion of other professions. The literature highlights two key features. First, the relationship is inherently unequal since the health professional has greater knowledge and authority over healthcare resources than the patient. Second, the health professional–patient relationship is, typically, involuntary and random. Often patients are assigned or choose their health professional based on health insurance coverage and availability when the patient is ill, rather than any personal qualities (Brown, Noble, Papageorgiou, & Kidd, 2016).

The health professions' literature rarely mentions interdependence and mutuality. When there is mention, it is typically in the context of professional-to-professional interactions and team-based care. Discussion of health professional–patient mutuality in the clinical setting is largely confined to both parties having a common goal, namely improving the patient's well-being. Assessment of mutuality in the clinical setting is limited to outcomes such as patient adherence to treatment protocols, patient understanding of their disease, patient coping skills, and patient satisfaction with the care they received. With psychiatry and nursing as the notable exceptions, the literature ignores the influence of mutuality with the patient on the health professional. This is an oversight. Anecdotal evidence of our bidirectional and interdependent relationship abounds, and is a prevalent theme expressed by our health professional colleagues who are also literary artists (Aronson, 2013; Campo, 2013; Ofri, 2003; Remen, 1996).

In this chapter, I aim to clarify the linkages among interdependence and clinical care. I summarize the literature on interdependence and mutuality from two fields: dialogic philosophy and Buddhist practice. I draw from the work of Martin Buber and Thich Nhat Hanh, and translate these teachings to the clinical setting. I review scholarly literature about health professional–patient dialogue and interpersonal relations, and consider what we can learn from our colleagues in psychiatry and nursing. I look at some of the opportunities for personal growth that derive from interdependent relationships in healthcare. The chapter concludes with exercises that stimulate experiential learning and deep engagement with mutuality and the interdependence of our relationships.

THOUGHTS ON INTERDEPENDENCE AND MUTUALITY

Two fields have mature, scholarly discourse on interdependence and mutuality that readily link to clinical care: dialogic philosophy, specifically the work of Martin Buber; and the Buddhist idea of interbeing as expressed by Zen master teacher and peace activist, Thich Nhat Hanh. Certainly, other fields and scholars have explored the idea of interdependent relationships. I deliberately chose the literature for this chapter based on its direct applicability to clinical practice.

DIALOGIC PHILOSOPHY – MARTIN BUBER

In 1923 scholar and philosopher, Martin Buber, published the text, *I and Thou*, thus launching the field of dialogic philosophy (Buber, 2000). I provide a brief summary of Buber's premise about how humans engage with each other. I strongly urge you to read *I and Thou* to fully appreciate the poetic brilliance of Buber's writing and experience his argument for relationship with non-human entities.

Martin Buber describes two ways by which we relate to the world around us: "I and It" versus "I and Thou." In the "I and It" relationship, I objectify It – even when It is another person. I view It as a collection of distinct qualities and attributes for my use, to satisfy my needs, to help me achieve my goal. I analyze It rather than fully recognizing the totality of the person's presence. At its most flagrant, the objectification that occurs in an "I and It" relationship is the basis for misogyny, racism, and exploitation. Yet when we look closely, we see how easily objectification creeps into our encounters even when we are not overtly discriminatory. In clinical care, this happens when we think of our patients as simply their diagnoses, at the exclusion of their personhood. While the days of crassly referring to patients as "the hip fracture in room 4" are nearly extinct, it is still common, in our devotion to expediency, to catalogue people exclusively by their biomedical frame. In doing so, we limit them to a problem that we can fix, thereby satisfying our professional need to achieve competence. However, we must consider what gets lost in the process. Our humanity dwindles each time we objectify another person, and the possibility for our own growth is thwarted.

Now let's look at the richness that "I and Thou" engagement offers us, both personally and professionally. The "I and Thou" encounter expects both parties are active participants in the relationship. Thou recognizes I and I recognizes Thou as an entirety, a person with a totality of experience, a manifestation of the universe – rather than a collection of qualities and attributes. When I and Thou meet, the relationship itself is transformative. In the text, *Martin Buber's Narrow Ridge and the Human Sciences*, philosopher Maurice Friedman (1996, p. 18) provides insight into the expansive nature of the "I and Thou" relationship and the role "I and It" relationship plays in bringing "I and Thou" to fruition.

> Starting with the philosophy of dialogue, we can say that the I-Thou relation is a direct knowing that gives one neither knowledge about the Thou over against the I nor about oneself as an objective entity apart from that relationship. . . . Although this dialogical knowing is direct, it is not entirely unmediated. The directness of the relationship is established not only through the mediation of the senses in the concrete meeting of real living persons, but also through mediation of the word. That means the mediation of those fields of symbolic communication, such as language, music, art, and ritual, which enable human beings ever again to enter into relation with what comes to meet them. The word may be identified with subject-object or I-It knowledge while it remains indirect and symbolic. However, it is itself the channel of expression of I-Thou knowing when it is taken up into real dialogue.

When we elevate our relationships to "I and Thou" encounters, dialogue is the unifying agent that helps us understand and reveal ourselves to each other. "The meaning of this dialogue is found in neither one nor the other of the partners, nor in both added together, but in their interchange" (Friedman, 1983, p. 6). When I and Thou contribute authentically to the dialogue, a potent transformation can occur for both. Authentic contribution demands the presence of our true self, and cannot arise when we subsume our identity to our professional roles (see chapter 9 Professional Identity: Perspectives, Roles, Values, and Attributes). When two self-aware and attentive humans meet, the encounter is intimate.

MUTUALITY AND ONE-SIDED RELATIONSHIPS

In clinical care, is it possible to maintain our professional boundaries and ethical practice and still allow for the intimacy of "I and Thou" engagement with patients? Martin Buber wrote a postscript to *I and Thou* which asserts the answer is yes – to a degree. Buber sequesters one-sided relationships, specifically identifying teacher–student, physician–patient, and clergy–congregant dyads as problematic. Buber states mutuality can be present in these relationships; however, it cannot achieve its full influence because of the constraints imposed by the professional role and obligation to carry out a task.

> Genuine learning, healing, and forgiving occur only in the noninstrumentality and acceptance of the I-Thou relation. But the pupil, the patient, and the penitent each has a need, arrangements for the meeting of which introduce elements which qualify not only mutuality but also each of the other basic characteristics of relation.
>
> (Berry, 1985, p. 52)

Colgate University professor and Episcopal priest, Donald L. Berry, explores Buber's argument that mutuality must be incomplete because of the one-sided, normative limitations of professional relationships. In the book, *Mutuality: The Vision of Martin Buber*, Professor Berry (1985) systematically dismantles the parameters of Buber's argument and ultimately extends Buber's vision to include the learning, healing, and forgiving relationships. Berry confirms there are limits on mutuality imposed by the professional task; however, he moves our thinking further by allowing the mutuality of the interpersonal relation to continue *beyond* the professional task.

> we may describe these relationships as coming into being and persisting so long as the task or purpose defines the contact. Relation, on the other hand, is a possible aspect of such continuing purposive relationships. The one-sidedness of the helping relationship does not, in principle, have to extend in the same way to the relation itself. Indeed, the goal is to humanize the relationships in the I-Thou attitude, to permeate all relationships with relation.
>
> (p. 66)

In other words, the professional relationship and its obligatory tasks exist within the generous expanse of two humans, undifferentiated by role, providing mutual recognition and presence.

It may be helpful to step out of the clinical setting to find further support for the existence of an interdependent relationship with unequal knowledge and authority. Let's look at a relationship that is familiar to many of us: parent and young child. Whether you have been a parent, a child, or both, you most likely will agree that there is an inherent skew in knowledge and authority toward the parent. The parent, generally speaking, knows how to navigate the world to keep the child safe, and controls access to life-sustaining resources like food, water, and shelter. The young child is dependent on the parent for physical and emotional care and guidance. At first glance, this looks like a one-sided relationship. When we look more deeply, we see that for the parent the relationship with the young child offers the opportunity to reignite curiosity, joy, awe, and unconditional love. It is a chance to see the world in a fresh, new way. In a healthy parent–child relationship, interdependence and mutuality are undeniable.

With the ideas of dialogic philosophy and intimate engagement in mind, let's continue the discussion of interdependence through the Buddhist philosophy lens.

BUDDHIST PRACTICE – THICH NHAT HANH

Buddhism presents interdependent nature as an experience of reality that one can have by concentrating deeply on an object (including a person) to see wholly into the nature of that object (Emmanuel, 2013). Unlike other concepts in Buddhism, interdependent nature is not a philosophical argument, but rather an invitation to use our personal encounters to understand our world and ourselves. In his text, *The Miracle of Mindfulness*, Zen master teacher, author, and peace activist, Thich Nhat Hanh (1975, p. 70) introduces interdependent nature by relating subject of knowledge and object of knowledge.

> To see is to see something. To hear is to hear something. To be angry is to be angry over something. Hope is hope for something. Thinking is thinking about something. When the object of knowledge (the something) is not present, there can be no subject of knowledge. The practitioner meditates on mind and, by so doing, is able to see the interdependence of the subject of knowledge and the object of knowledge.

Thich Nhat Hanh highlights the interdependent nature of our experiences, perceptions, and cognitions, which in turn feed our interdependence with others. The following sections continue our exploration of interdependent nature.

FIVE AGGREGATES

In preparation for more in-depth discussion of interdependence, I list here the five aggregates of Buddhist philosophy, also called the objects of mind: bodily and physical forms, feelings, perceptions, mental functionings, and consciousness. Consciousness is understood to be the basis for the other four aggregates (Emmanuel, 2013). The five aggregates are impermanent, continually evolving elements that make up each of us. I encourage you to take a moment to observe the five aggregates in yourself. As you do so, notice how each aggregate only exists in relationship to the world beyond you. I share with you my observations while contemplating the five aggregates: My bodily form is tailored to the physical environment and is dependent upon water, air, gravity, and food external to my body to survive. The performance capacity of my bodily form also depends on my surroundings: If I breathe polluted air, I may experience respiratory distress; if I eat tainted and/or nutrient-depleted food, I likely suffer the consequences of infectious disease and malnutrition; if I have inadequate shelter leading to prolonged exposure to extreme weather conditions, my physical abilities quickly become impaired. My feelings, perceptions, and mental functionings exist so I can process, catalog, interpret, and understand the world around me. For example, I may feel anger toward someone, derived from my perception of threat, which evolves from my memory of past threats to my well-being. While transient and mutable, my feelings, perceptions, and mental functionings are also unique to me and arise from my prior experiences, socialization, and habits of mind.

My consciousness exists solely because I have something of which to be conscious. Based on my personal observations, I am able to see the five aggregates develop from the world, moment by moment, and I resonate with Thich Nhat Hanh's (1975, p. 74) statement,

> The self is no different from the assembly of the five aggregates themselves. The assembly of the five aggregates plays, as well, a crucial role in the formation, creation, and destruction of all things in the universe.

Again, this is not a philosophy to be argued or a doctrine to be swallowed; this is simply an experience that you may or may not share.

MINDFULNESS

To cultivate the experience of interdependence, you may wish to explore the practice of mindfulness. At this time in the Western hemisphere, the word mindfulness is ubiquitous, largely rendering it devoid of precise meaning. For the purpose of our discussion, I rely on the definition of mindfulness provided by Thich Nhat Hanh, "keeping one's consciousness alive to the present reality" (Nhat Hanh, 1975, p. 16). By this definition, mindfulness does not require sequestered space, ability to hold a physical posture, or even quiet. The only requirement is that we levy open awareness and concentration on the object of our attention – be it a person, thing, or task. This means we can practice mindfulness throughout our day, whether we are brushing our teeth, cooking, walking the hospital corridor, interviewing a patient, suturing or dressing a wound, performing cardiopulmonary resuscitation, or sitting in silence.

> There is no reason why mindfulness should be different from focusing all one's attention on one's work, to be alert and to be using one's best judgment. During the moment one is consulting, resolving, and dealing with whatever arises, a calm heart and self-control are necessary if one is to obtain good results.
>
> (p. 20)

I invite you to experiment with bringing mindfulness to your everyday life. Pick one task that you do routinely, for example, walking from the classroom to the cafeteria, the bus stop to the hospital, or your car to the clinic. During the few moments when you walk to your destination, bring your attention to your feet on the floor or ground, the transfer of your weight from one leg to the other, the ambient air on your skin as you move through space, and the light meeting your eyes. Fully experience moving your physical body from point A to point B, and note how that experience differs from when you stride between places lost in thought – recounting diagnostic studies you need to order, the consultation request you need to write, and the groceries you need to buy. Notice if applying mindful attention affects your stamina, mood, relationships with your patients, and/or other aspects of your life. The experiment is yours to conduct. The experience is yours to have.

Thich Nhat Hanh (1975, 2006) teaches the transformative capacity of mindfulness practice. Mindfulness allows us to recognize when a negative habit of mind (e.g., anger, discrimination, jealousy, despair) arises, and tenderly embrace the negative habit of mind (as opposed to suppressing or pushing it away), so we can look deeply at the negative habit of mind and the root conditions that contribute to its existence. When we concentrate our attention to look deeply at the nature of our negative habit of mind, there is opportunity for insight. Insight can transform our negative habit of mind and liberate us from its alienating clutches. Once liberated, we are able to appreciate the concept of interbeing, which I discuss next.

INTERBEING

Several decades ago, Thich Nhat Hanh coined the term interbeing, which he derived from the Mahayana School of Buddhism Avatamsaka Sutra. Interbeing is the idea that if we are to be, to exist, we must be mutual with others. Thich Nhat Hanh (1987, p. 88) writes,

> We have talked about the many in the one, and the one containing the many.
> In one sheet of paper, we see everything else, the cloud, the forest, the logger.
> I am, therefore you are. You are, therefore I am. That is the meaning of the word
> interbeing. We interare.

For many years now, I have hung a sign in my office with Thich Nhat Hanh's words, "I am, therefore you are. You are, therefore I am." I regularly reflect on these subtle, powerful, and humbling words. The idea that our relationships are the substrate from which we emerge as individuals and influence each other definitely gives me pause. When I feel alienated by a colleague, frustrated by a student, or aggravated by a patient, if I recall the statement, "I am, therefore you are. You are, therefore I am," then I am motivated to explore my contribution to the negative emotions. With awareness, I have the opportunity to transform my negative emotions into something more wholesome that can favorably influence the encounter. It does not come naturally or easily to me, however, when I bring attention to the encounter and plod my way to awareness, I am able to experience a positive shift for myself and the other person involved.

The implications for interbeing in healthcare are many. Let's start by looking at identity. Our identity as a health professional is predicated on the presence of a patient. Our purpose as health professionals is to care for patients. Despite the fact that our days may be laden with non-patient care tasks, our raison d'etre as nurse, PA, physician, social worker, psychologist, physical therapist, or any other health professional is to care for patients. Similarly, someone is not a patient unless he seeks care from a health professional – until then he is a person who is ill or injured. When we acknowledge the interbeing of health professional and patient, then we can focus on the relationship and let go of perceptions such as vulnerable person, authority figure, helper, and recipient (see chapter 8 Uncertainty and Decision Making). In a similar vein, awareness of interbeing makes it impossible for us to hold discriminatory or biased perspectives of our patients.

Thich Nhat Hanh (2006, p. 210) writes, "When we stop and look deeply into our mental formations, our notions of self and other, birth and death, ignorance and awakening, then we see their true self-nature of interdependence. That is interbeing." If we do not see the patient as "other" but rather see the patient and ourselves as complete, interconnected manifestations of the world, then our natural inclination is therapeutic caring. When the relationship has primacy, the encounter liberates us to grow beyond our tasks and responsibilities to co-create the world.

HEALTH PROFESSIONAL–PATIENT RELATIONSHIPS AND DIALOGUE

Health professional–patient communication has been a topic of research for decades. The existing literature is vast and covers issues as far-reaching as establishing rapport to facilitating health behavior change to cross-cultural awareness. It is important and interesting work that continues to inform the effective delivery of healthcare. Amid the mountain of data and opinion about health professional–patient communication, there exists a small body of literature on dialogue and relationships. This is where I will focus the next part of the discussion of interdependence and mutuality.

THEORY OF HUMAN CARING

Distinguished professor of nursing and dean emerita at the University of Colorado, and founder and director of the Watson Caring Science Institute, Jean Watson, PhD, RN, FAAN (1997), developed and refined the Theory of Human Caring. Professor Watson originally developed the theory to bring meaning and distinction to professional nursing practice. Over the years, the Theory of Human Caring led to scientific inquiry of caring, which has evolved to become a transdisciplinary field with general relevance to healthcare and human service. Within the Theory of Human Caring, Professor Watson (2008) provides seven core concepts that demonstrate interdependence and mutuality. The core concepts are:

1   the relationship is the basis for caring for self and others;
2   caring relationships transcend the interpersonal;
3   caring encounters lead to heightened awareness for self and other;
4   there are multiple ways of knowing;
5   reflection increases consciousness and awareness of self and other;
6   caring is inclusive of self, other, environment, and universe; and
7   caring changes self, other, and the larger culture.

Professor Watson (1997, p. 50) writes that these core concepts are "those aspects of nursing that actually potentiate therapeutic healing processes and relationships; they affect the one caring and the-one-being-cared for." As the seven concepts demonstrate, the Theory of Human Caring and caring science are fundamentally relational. They allow the activity of caring to be a conduit for expanded consciousness for the health professional, patient, family, and society.

INTERACTION ADAPTATION THEORY

The Interaction Adaptation Theory posits that when two people are talking, communication patterns change for each member of the dyad depending on whether one's needs are met by the other member of the dyad (Burgoon, Stern, & Dillman, 1995). When there is mutual influence among the dyad members, they achieve reciprocity in their communication patterns. This means the communication pattern of each member grows in similarity to the communication pattern of the other member. In contrast, when there is unidirectional influence, typically one member of the dyad having power over the other, their communication patterns reveal compensation. This means the dyad members diverge or become more dissimilar in their expressed communication patterns over time.

Based on the Interaction Adaptation Theory, researchers designed a study to examine the expression of relationship-centered care in clinical practice through health professional–patient communication patterns. The authors describe relationship-centered care in terms consistent with interdependence and mutuality.

> Relationship-centered care recognizes the personhood of both participants, acknowledges the importance of affect and emotion, places all healthcare relationships in the context of reciprocal influence, and infers moral value on the formation and maintenance of genuine relationships in healthcare.
> (Duggan & Bradshaw, 2008, p. 212)

The researchers videotaped patient encounters and then coded non-verbal behaviors and verbal expressions from both the patient and health professional. Their analysis revealed evidence of mutual influence, in the form of reciprocal expression, for non-verbal behaviors such as smiling and nodding. In contrast, there was evidence of unidirectional influence, in the form of compensation, for breaking eye contact, verbal dysfluency, and discussion about barriers to wellness. The split between mutual influence for non-verbal expression and unidirectional influence for verbal expression reminds me of research on non-verbal behaviors and the unconscious mind (Pally, 2001). If we accept that non-verbal behaviors are more highly associated with our unconscious awareness than verbal expression is, then we can postulate that our unconscious intention as health professionals and patients is to achieve mutual influence. However, before we achieve mutual influence, our verbal expression, guided by our rigid interpretation of roles and responsibilities, tugs us toward compensation and one-sided influence. Obviously, this postulate is outside the interpretive range of this single study; it is, however, impetus for future research.

SHARED PRESENCE

Recent research on shared presence helps to advance our understanding of interdependence and mutuality during the healthcare encounter. Health professional communication scholars, William Ventres, MD and Richard Frankel, PhD (2015, p. 272), describe shared presence as "a state of being in which physicians and other health professionals and their patients enter into a deep sense of trust, respect, and knowing that facilitates healing." Ventres and Frankel acknowledge that shared presence is rare in clinical care, and that it occurs within the milieu of routine health professional–patient communication. With the aim of recognizing and cultivating shared presence, Ventres and Frankel set out to conceptualize the necessary conditions for shared presence to materialize. They synthesized multiple theories of health professional communication and empirical evidence of deeply satisfying, emotionally connected, and mutually beneficial patient encounters to arrive at four elemental factors associated with shared presence. Three of the four factors, interpersonal skills, relational contexts, and actions in the patient encounters, contribute to shared presence; the fourth factor, healing outcomes, is a consequence of shared presence. Here is a brief description of each of the factors.

The specific interpersonal skills Ventres and Frankel distill for us are self-awareness, awareness of the patient, curiosity, and being open to other perspectives – all with the goal of encountering the patient as a human being with inimitable qualities, attributes, and responses to illness. Relational context refers to the clinical integration of the patient's psychological health, social environment, and spiritual beliefs. As discussed in chapter 2 Patient as Storyteller, cultural and psychosocial determinants can have a profound impact on the patient's well-being. When we include these aspects of the patient's world in the clinical encounter, we not only see potential challenges to care but also receive a clear view of the patient as a whole person with appreciable strengths. Ventres and Frankl describe the third factor contributing to shared presence, actions in the patient encounter, as our habits of practice. This includes the uniquely personal ways that we, as individual health professionals, set up the clinical encounter to build rapport, demonstrate empathy, and motivate patients, while simultaneously conducting a biomedical assessment. The fourth factor, healing outcomes, is the product of shared presence and includes process outcomes as well as therapeutic outcomes. The process outcomes relate to interdependence and mutuality. "Process outcomes are mutual emotional sentiments, experienced by both patients and physicians. They include intimacy, partnership, understanding, and trust" (Ventres & Frankel, 2015, p. 274). Furthermore, the favorable process outcomes constructively influence therapeutic outcomes such as treatment adherence and follow-up care. Consistent with the concept of interbeing and Theory of Human Caring (described earlier), shared presence offers the opportunity for clinician and patient to transcend the confines of roles and meet as human beings.

EXTRAORDINARY CLINICIANS

Vanderbilt University professors, David Schenck and Larry Churchill (2012), conducted an ethnographic study of "extraordinary clinicians." Their aim was to discern the composition of healing relationships and the means by which health professionals learn to become healers, not simply technicians. Professors Schenck and Churchill conducted face-to-face interviews with 50 clinicians who were identified by their peers as being able to establish and maintain excellent relationships with patients. They asked the clinicians a series of open-ended, semi-structured questions in four topic areas: establishing relationships, how healing happens, experiences as a patient, and self-care. The entire book is fascinating. Most relevant to this chapter on interdependence is the section on self-care. When the clinicians were asked about activities they personally engage in to promote wellness, wholeness, and healing, a number of clinicians referred to their patients as a resource. The clinicians said their patients "were often a source of renewal and healing for them." One clinician described "being carried in the healing energy that patients bring with them"; others spoke of "the privilege of being in the presence of people who could mobilize their own healing resources" (p 169). By being present and attentive to themselves and their patients, these clinicians were able to recognize the patients' contributions to the relationship and thrive on the virtues of engagement.

OPPORTUNITIES FOR PERSONAL GROWTH

The health professions are rich with opportunities for personal growth. Many of us are attracted to the health professions because the frontier of biomedical knowledge is continually extending into new territory. The challenge and thrill of life-long learning provides fertile ground for intellectual growth and skill building. The focus of this chapter on interdependence and mutuality points toward another avenue for personal growth, namely expansion of our understanding of self and the world we live in. At first glance, it seems counterintuitive that engaging with someone who is debilitated may lead to our personal growth. We value wholeness, health, and independence, so why would we deliberately link ourselves to someone with a physical and/or psychological limitation – especially someone who is a relative stranger? By bringing our full self into relationship with the patient, we have the potential to experience a wisdom and meaning that is typically inaccessible to those without disease (Frank, 2013). By working with patients from cultural and social groups other than those we are familiar with, we learn the many ways illness can alter one's self-perception and identity, reorder one's priorities, and demand that we traverse the rugged territory of loneliness, uncertainty, loss, and grief. These are gifts, life lessons that come from being open to an interdependent relationship with our patients.

HEALTH PROFESSIONAL EDUCATION

Let's turn our attention to health professional education. Our professional education drills us on "standards" so that all of our patients receive the highest possible level of care. We have "professional standards," "standards of care," and "performance standards." We are taught to think in a particular way to systematically arrive at a diagnosis, to maneuver in a precise manner to elicit physical examination signs and execute procedures, and to communicate using meticulous language – all of which elevates our ability to provide excellent healthcare. Great news, right? Unfortunately, the educational process may also homogenize us, in effect dismantling the exquisite self we could bring to our relationships with patients. While we embrace standards for quality, ethical care, we must simultaneously defy the homogenization of our personhood. We are not interchangeable. Who we are as individuals has healing power, because our presence has healing power, and our presence is only possible when we bring our whole self to the relationship.

By recognizing our interdependence and mutuality, and increasing our self-awareness, health professionals step onto a pathway to clinical care that allows us to maintain our humanity and develop our wisdom.

PSYCHIATRY

Our colleagues in psychiatry and nursing have shown greater inclination to acknowledge interdependence and mutuality with patients than those of us in other health professions. I described nursing's Theory of Human Caring earlier. Here I provide input from psychiatry.

In 2018, the *Creative Practice as Mutual Recovery* (CPMR) program completed five years of research in the United Kingdom, United States, China, and Spain focused on determining the effect of shared creative practices on patients, family members, and health professionals (Crawford et al., 2018). The aim of the CPMR research team was to examine mutuality and "mutual recovery" among individuals with a mental health diagnosis and the professionals and family members who cared for them, using creative practices "to establish and connect communities" (p. 5). Under the auspices of the CPMR program, a total of 14 projects were completed. The research team writes,

> The CPMR programme found compelling and substantial quantitative and qualitative evidence for the benefits of diverse shared creative practices in generating "mutual recovery" of mental health and well-being both within and between different groups of people in different social and professional roles.
>
> (p. 3)

CPMR was the first large scale initiative to use creative practices to look at mutuality and interdependence among patients and health professionals. Before widespread integration of creative practices like those tested in CPMR will occur, there will need to be policy and infrastructure changes in healthcare. I encourage you to visit the digital showcase of the CPMR projects (http://cpmr.mentalhealth.org.uk/). Perhaps you will find inspiration for mutuality programming and/or research that you can conduct at your institution.

The late Yale University professor and physician, Hans Loewald, MD (1980, p. 297) wrote,

> To discover truth about the patient is always discovering it with him and for him as well as for ourselves and about ourselves. And it is discovering truth between each other, as the truth of human beings is revealed in their interrelatedness.

It is easy to dismiss this approach as bound to the paradigms of transference and countertransference that form the basis of psychiatric care, and therefore have little applicability to other disciplines. I believe this is a mistake. Dr. Loewald and others emphasize the distinct and reciprocal nature of the relationship, and the healing effect patients can have on the health professional.

In the text, *Power in the Helping Professions*, psychotherapist Adolf Guggenbuhl-Craig (1971, p. 130) speaks of the way his patients illuminate his own issues. He writes, the attentive and receptive therapist "recognizes time and again how the patient's difficulties constellate his own problems and vice versa, and he therefore openly works not only on the patient, but on himself. He remains forever a patient as well as a healer." As with any human-to-human interaction, if we are open and receptive to our patients, we have the opportunity to learn and grow from the potent, bidirectional influence of the relationship.

CLOSING

In this chapter, we looked at the linkages among interdependence, mutuality, and clinical care. We reviewed the literature on interdependence and mutuality from dialogic philosophy and Buddhist practice, and translated these teachings to the clinical setting. We looked at scholarly endeavors about health professional–patient dialogue and interpersonal relations. Finally, we highlighted some of the opportunities for personal growth that derive from interdependent relationships in healthcare.

I close this chapter with learning objectives and activities that provide the reader with the opportunity to explore the interdependence and mutuality present in our personal and professional relationships.

ACTIVITIES

LEARNING OBJECTIVES

Learners will

1 explore the potential for interdependence within the health professional–patient relationship;
2 reflect on their personal experience of interdependent relationships.

BOOK EXCERPT AND DISCUSSION

First, read the excerpt entitled, *Stage 2 Chapter 17 Tumor Board* pp. 113–115, from the book, *Bright Hour: A Memoir of Living and Dying*, by Nina Riggs (2017). As you read, note words or passages that appeal to you, repel you, resonate with you, startle you, or in some way catch your attention. Drawing on material presented in chapter 6, reflect on the interdependence and mutuality among the characters in the chapter.

SMALL GROUP DISCUSSION

Learners are invited to discuss their experience with the chapter. Whenever possible, learners should refer to specific passages in the chapter. In particular, learners should aim to comment on interdependent relationships. Faculty facilitators may choose to ask someone to read aloud a passage from the story that captured their attention. Reading aloud makes the text a presence in the room and helps everyone focus. If at all possible, allow the conversation about the text to evolve organically, directed by the learners' curiosity.

NOTE: **Appendix A** has general guidelines for facilitating a health humanities seminar. **Appendix B** has instruction and discussion prompts specific to this activity for faculty facilitators to use if your learners are not able to initiate a robust discussion.

WRITING AND SHARING

The second activity is for the learner to write to a prompt that directly links the content of this chapter and the book excerpt. Here is a suggested writing prompt:

> Write about a time you were ". . . in the middle of six lanes of a chaotic highway, but tucked inside the pod of a tollbooth." Feel free to write fiction.

Faculty facilitators can invite the learners to share what they have written with the group. Learners should never be required to share their writings.

REFERENCE LIST

Aronson, L. (2013). *A history of present illness*. New York: Bloomsbury.

Berry, D. L. (1985). *Mutuality: The vision of Martin Buber*. Albany, NY: State University of New York.

Brown, J., Noble, L. M., Papageorgiou, A., & Kidd, J. (Eds.). (2016). *Clinical communication in medicine*. West Sussex, UK: Wiley-Blackwell.

Buber, M. (2000). *I and Thou*. Translated by R. G. Smith. New York: Scribner Classics.

Burgoon, J. K., Stern, L. A., & Dillman, L. (1995). *Interpersonal adaptation*. New York: Cambridge University Press.

Campo, R. (2013). *Alternative medicine*. Durham, NC: Duke University Press.

Crawford, P., Hogan, S., Wilson, M., Williamon, A., Manning, N., Brown, B., & Lewis, L. (2018). *Creative practice as mutual recovery: Research programme final*

report. University of Nottingham: UK, China, Malaysia. Retrieved from www.
healthhumanities.org/documents/Creative-Practice-as-Mutual-Recovery-Final-
Report-20180412.pdf

Duggan, A. P., & Bradshaw, Y. S. (2008). Mutual influence processes in physician-
patient communication: An interaction adaptation perspective. *Communication
Research Reports, 25*(3), 211–226.

Emmanuel, S. M. (Ed.). (2013). *A companion to Buddhist philosophy*. West Sussex,
UK: Wiley-Blackwell.

Frank, A. (2013). *The wounded storyteller: Body, illness, and ethics* (2nd ed.).
Chicago, IL: University of Chicago Press.

Friedman, M. (1983). *The confirmation of otherness in family, community, and
society*. New York: Pilgrim.

Friedman, M. (1996). Martin Buber's narrow ridge and the human sciences. In M.
Friedman, P. Boni, L. Baron, S. Cain, V. Shabatay, & J. Stewart (Eds.), *Martin Buber
and the human sciences*. Albany, NY: State University of New York.

Guggenbuhl-Craig, A. (1971). *Power in the helping professions*. New York: Spring.

Loewald, H. W. (1980). *Papers on psychoanalysis*. New Haven, CT: Yale University
Press.

Nhat Hanh, T. (1975). *The miracle of mindfulness*. Boston, MA: Beacon.

Nhat Hanh, T. (1987). *Being peace*. Berkeley, CA: Parallax.

Nhat Hanh, T. (2006). *Understanding our mind*. Berkeley, CA: Parallax.

Ofri, D. (2003). *Singular intimacies: Becoming a doctor at Bellevue*. New York:
Penguin.

Pally, R. (2001). A primary role for nonverbal communication in psychoanalysis.
Psychoanalytic Inquiry, 21(1), 7193.

Remen, R. N. (1996). *Kitchen table wisdom: Stories that heal*. New York: Riverhead
Books.

Riggs, N. (2017). *Bright hour: A memoir of living and dying*. New York: Simon and
Schuster.

Schenck, D., & Churchill, L. (2012). *Healers: Extraordinary clinicians at work*. New
York: Oxford University Press.

Ventres, W. B., & Frankel, R. M. (2015). Shared presence in physician-patient communication: A graphic representation. *Families, Systems, & Health, 33*(3), 270–279.

Watson, J. (1997). The theory of human caring: Retrospective and prospective. *Nursing Science Quarterly, 10*(1), 49–52.

Watson, J. (2008). *Nursing: The philosophy and science of caring, revised edition.* Boulder, CO: University Press of Colorado.

7 THE INFLUENCE OF TIME ON MEANING

INTEGRATION NOTE
....
This chapter integrates with clinical science content on cancer care and chronic disease management, as well as instruction about family caregivers and the effect of disease on family units. It also complements material on health professional well-being.

INTRODUCTION

Time is a powerful actor in clinical care for both health professionals and patients. For health professionals, the objective measure of time is a formidable opponent in a continuous game of Beat the Clock. Whether our aim is to see a patient every 10 minutes in an outpatient clinic, manage an inpatient service, insert an endotracheal tube expediently, or change intravenous lines to mitigate risk of infection, time often dictates our perceptions and actions in the clinical setting. For patients, the metric of time is important, however, the subjective experience of time poses the greater challenge. From the moment one assumes the role of patient, time is a factor. At one extreme, time passes slowly as patients wait for appointments, wait for biopsy results, and wait for pain medication to "kick in." At another extreme, patients experience the acceleration of time conferred by a life-altering diagnosis. The goal of this chapter is to look at the influence of time on the meaning we can derive from health and illness. Therefore, I focus most of our attention on subjective time and largely set aside the conversation about objective time. In healthcare, the issues associated with the objective measure of time are primarily a systems-level problem that is beyond the scope of this chapter. That said, the pervasive presence of objective time issues in healthcare means objective time is invariably part of our discussion.

It is important to note that there is not a coherent theory of time. More than 1,600 years ago, St. Augustine (2014, Book XI, Chapter XIV) wrote,

> What then is time? If no one asks me, I know what it is. If I wish to explain it to him who asks, I do not know. Yet I say with confidence, that I know that if nothing passed away, there would not be past time; and if nothing were coming, there would not be future time; and if nothing were, there would not be present time. Those two times, therefore, past and future, how are they, when even the past now is not; and the future is not as yet? But should the present be always present, and should it not pass into time past, time truly it could not be, but eternity. If, then, time present – if it be time – only comes into existence because it passes into time past, how do we

say that even this is, whose cause of being is that it shall not be – namely, so that we cannot truly say that time is, unless because it tends not to be?

Perhaps St. Augustine expresses time as a riddle, at least in part because the multidimensional nature of time and the ambiguity of many of its qualities make the confines of a definition fragile. Modern day thinkers about time are similarly challenged. For example, some of the ancient debates remain relevant in modern times, specifically: Can physical, objective time be reconciled with subjective time? Is story a mechanism for humans to capture and qualify our lived experience, despite (or perhaps because of) the unrelenting progression of physical time? How does our appreciation for past and future events affect our notion of ethical responsibility? (International Society for the Study of Time, n.d.). Thankfully, St. Augustine persevered beyond his earlier, oft-quoted statement, continued his rigorous study of time, and left a nuanced body of work for modern philosophers, as well as psychologists and physicists, to build upon. Over nearly two millennia, many great minds have dedicated themselves to demystifying the concept, which will make our discussion less about philosophical thought exercises and more about the grand influence that subjective time exerts on the illness narrative.

In this chapter, I explore the enigmatic concept of time from two fields: philosophy and cognitive science. Then I investigate the influence of time on patients' and health professionals' understanding of health and illness, the meaning we ascribe to our personal and sociocultural illness narrative, and the changes that meaning endures over time. The chapter concludes with reading and writing activities to stimulate experiential learning and personal engagement with the influence of time on meaning.

THOUGHTS ON TIME

For a preview of some of the dimensions of time, let's look at the variety of ways the word time is used in the English language, indicating a plethora of attributes.

FIGURES OF SPEECH

There are notable figures of speech in the English language that might lend insight into some of the Western cultural interpretations of time (Crystal, 2002). For example, we say, "Time flies." "Time stood still." "Time waits for no man." "Time heals all wounds." In these phrases, time has agency and asserts control.

We "kill" time. Prisoners are "doing" time. There are circumstances under which we can "make" time, "buy" time, "borrow" time, and "spend" time. In these phrases, *we* have the agency and time is the object of our actions: killing, doing, making, buying, borrowing, and spending.

Ben Franklin tells us, "Lost time is never found again" and "Time is money." With these two quotes, Franklin indicates time is a commodity, an entity with tradeable value.

Time as agent, time as object of action, and time as commodity – English language speakers do not allow this much flexibility for many other words. With this rich and varied parlance in mind, in the next sections I review some of the philosophical and cognitive science perspectives on time that directly relate to clinical care, in order to build a foundation for our discussion about the influence of time on one's ability to derive meaning from illness.

PHILOSOPHY OF TIME

Philosophy of time is a vast field. Here I present a few philosophical arguments that I feel are most helpful to our consideration of the influence of time on our interpretation of illness. As discussed in chapter 1 Introduction: The Power of Story, Explanatory Model of Disease section, culture influences one's interpretation of illness. Similarly, culture influences one's understanding of the concept of time. Therefore, I encourage you to explore philosophical perspectives on time for the patient culture groups you serve.

REALIST, RELATIONAL, AND IDEALIST VIEW OF TIME

Professor of Philosophy at Bradford University, Freidel Weinert (2013), in his book, *The March of Time: Evolving Conceptions of Time in the Light of Scientific Discoveries*, describes three categories of philosophy of time, namely the realist view, the relational view, and the idealist view. The realist view looks at time as a physical property of the universe. The "universe has a clock" per se that measures the progression of time, independent of other events. The relational view, developed by G. W. Leibniz in the 17th century, states that time only exists because there is a succession of regular and periodic events, or changes, that allow us to interpret time as before, during, and after an event. "The relation between time and change is reciprocal: Without change, there can be no recognition of time; and without time, there can be no measurement of change" (Weinert, 2013, p. 9).

The idealist view, developed by Immanuel Kant in the 18th century, asserts that time is an illusion, a construct of the mind, existing only because of human perception. The idealist view closely aligns with the reflections of St. Augustine who recognizes the human mind as the metric of time. According to Augustine, the human mind is a measurement tool based on its ability to be aware of present events, anticipate future events, and remember past events (St. Augustine, 2014). Within the idealist view, Kant does not deny the presence and importance of physical time; however, he privileges human perception of time over objective measures. Kant's work provides the basis for the concept of human time.

HUMAN TIME

Human time relies on physiological arousal and memory, and is molded by psychological state and individual bias. Human time is the perceived duration of events that arises from the flow of ideas stimulated by sensations. This means human time is variable and in a constant state of fluctuation (Eagleman, 2008). The difficulty with studying human time as a philosopher is that it depends upon an individual's personal, and often private observations, thus making it difficult to measure and compare temporal events. One person's human time is exactly that – one person's human time (Weinert, 2013). As I discuss later in this chapter (see Fusion of Time, Mind and Body: Revisited section), the unique experience dictated by human time is precisely the active ingredient of meaning making and patient-centered care.

COGNITIVE SCIENCE

The past two decades have seen a surge in knowledge about cognitive neuroscience. Among the advances, there is recent research that provides substantive, biologically based evidence of how humans experience time (Wittman, 2016). Studies show that when humans perceive a threat, sense danger, or experience emotionally charged events, in conjunction with physiologic arousal, our subjective experience of time is prolonged as compared to when we feel calm, safe, and emotionally neutral (Droit-Volet & Gil, 2009; van Wassenhove, Wittman, Craig, & Paulus, 2011). Perhaps you have noticed the dilation of time when you have been in situations such as: seeing a truck speeding toward you, walking on a dark street in a strange city, witnessing the birth of a child, or arguing with your significant other. Time can also feel prolonged when we are bored or anticipating something or someone (Wittman, 2016).

TEMPORAL PERCEPTION

Although there is as of yet no universally accepted theory of temporal perception among cognitive scientists, it is widely understood that the subjective experience of time is individual and conditional, and that an individual's appreciation for past, present, and future circumstances will "change constantly in the course of life" (Wittman, 2016, p. 84). The idea that our subjective experience is in a constant state of flux is difficult for most of us to grasp. Instead, we often believe that what we are experiencing now, will persist unabated in exactly the same way, into the future. For example, when we are happy and satisfied in a new intimate relationship, we rarely envision a future where that same person betrays us. Similarly, when we are distraught from having been betrayed by an intimate partner, there is a period of time when we are certain we will never be able to trust another person again. Despite ongoing evidence that our subjective experience is impermanent, we tend to cling to the belief that our situation is intransient and will remain so over time (Halifax, 2008).

In addition to life course changes in our perception of time, we alter our perception depending on when, in relation to the event, the judgment about time is being made – prospectively or retrospectively (Droit-Volet & Gil, 2009). Prospective judgment happens while an event is unfolding. The person involved deliberately focuses attention on the passage of time during the event. For example, the patient who is disrobed, covered only by a flimsy examination gown, legs dangling uncomfortably off the side of the examination table, who is counting the elapsed time until the health professional enters the room, is engaged in prospective judgment. Her human time experience, influenced by physical discomfort, boredom, and irritation at being made to wait, is that time is passing very slowly. Retrospective judgments, as the name implies, occur after an event ends and rely on memory. Several hours later, when the patient just described is warmly dressed, sitting comfortably in her own home, and recalling her diagnosis, treatment regimen, and the compassionate and thorough care that she received, her memory of the wait time in the examination room disintegrates.

In order to describe our lived experience and perception of time, we must have self-consciousness – awareness of our bodily presence in time and space. As Marc Wittman (2016, p. 88) writes,

> Consciousness is tied to corporeality and temporality: I experience myself as existing with a body over time. . . . I experience myself now as an embodied entity, but I also experience myself as persisting in time, beyond the moment.

Our patient described earlier is aware of her bodily sensations when she is in the exam room as well as when she recalls the encounter from her home. She is self-cognizant in the present (while waiting) and in the past (while recollecting), and in different space dimensions (examination room and home). However, her perception of time duration and how she remembers her physical discomfort varies as her priorities shift during the passage of time – in this case, a matter of hours. In effect, her narrative of her experience changes over time because of the interplay of time, mind, and body. Time has passed and the patient's body has changed – from cold and uncomfortable in the examination room to warm and cozy at home; and her mind has changed – from bored and irritated in the exam room to intrigued by her diagnosis, hopeful about her treatment plan, and grateful for her care.

PAIN AND TEMPORAL PERCEPTION

Now let's consider what happens to temporality, corporeality, and self-consciousness in the presence of intractable pain. There is remarkably little research investigating time perception for individuals in pain. One qualitative study of patients with chronic, unyielding pain demonstrated that participants had a slowed perception of time (Thomas & Johnson, 2000). Drawing from an accumulation of anecdotal evidence found in patient biographies and the arts, Professor David Morris (2010, p. 52) writes,

> Intractable pain has an atypical time signature built into its structure. Its most alien feature, separating it from the familiar and somewhat reassuring model of acute pain, is the threat of endlessness: pain that never stops.

The danger of perceived endlessness, an infinite future filled with pain, is that the patient is now devoid of hope and bereft from a normal sense of self. Pain alienates us from our body and catches us in a warped time perception, thus compromising the influences among temporality, corporeality, and consciousness. Author and activist Audre Lorde (1997, p. 24) writes in her book, *The Cancer Journals,*

10/10/78 I want to write of the pain I am feeling right now, of the lukewarm tears that will not stop coming into my eyes – for what? For my lost breast? For the lost me? And which me was that again anyway? . . . I'm so tired of all this. I want to be the person I used to be, the real me. I feel sometimes that it's all a dream and surely I'm about to wake up now.

With this quote, Ms. Lorde captures the anguish and distortion pain imposes on her sense of time and self-awareness. Nineteen months later, Ms. Lorde (p. 12) writes

5/30/80 Last spring was another piece of the fall and winter before, a progression from all the pain and sadness of that time, ruminated over. But somehow this summer which is almost upon me feels like a part of my future. Like a brand new time, and I'm pleased to know it, wherever it leads.

In this second quote, Ms. Lorde has a decidedly different perception of time, as well as a changed physical and psychological relationship to time. The burdensome, interminable nature of time has lifted and been replaced by expectant curiosity. Pain – both psychic and physical – can seriously undermine our ability to make meaning of illness. This discussion continues in more detail later in the chapter in the section, Influence of Time on Our Understanding of Illness.

FUSION OF TIME, MIND, AND BODY

The fields of philosophy and cognitive science support the premise that for time to be perceived, one needs consciousness and corporeality, which we can also term mind and body. As humans, we braid time, mind, and body to create and understand our experience. Recall from chapter 1 the definition of disease, "abnormalities in the structure and function of body organs and systems," and illness, "experiences of disvalued changes in states of being and in social function; the human experience of sickness" (Kleinman, Eisenberg, & Good, 1978, p. 251). Disease and illness exist in comparison to a biologically normal state of being and perceived wellness – and by their very definitions, mandate the fusion of time, mind, and body. Passage of time must occur for one to transition from biologically, functionally, and perceptibly normal to abnormal – which brings us to the crux of this chapter: to ponder the influence time has on our ability to make meaning of illness.

INFLUENCE OF TIME ON OUR UNDERSTANDING OF ILLNESS

CANCER FAMILY CAREGIVER INTERVIEWS

A few years ago, colleagues and I conducted a research study of family caregivers to adults receiving active treatment for lung or colon cancer. One part of the study consisted of individual, face-to-face interviews with family caregivers, during which they talked about their experiences of caring for their ill family members (Williams & Bakitas, 2012). Almost without exception, their experiences and the meaning they were able to derive from their experiences varied over time from when they heard the diagnosis, to caring for their ill family member after surgery, to the period when the family member was receiving chemotherapy. Following are illustrative quotes from the caregivers about three phases during the illness: diagnosis, surgical aftermath, and chemotherapy. As you read the caregivers' words and interpret the meaning the caregivers created, consider the links among time, mind, and body. The caregiver's relationship to the patient is in brackets before each quote.

NEW DIAGNOSIS

At the time of a new cancer diagnosis, the dominant expressions for most people were shock, disbelief, fear, and uncertainty.

[father]   Well, the most immediate incident is knowing that he had cancer. It's like a bullet in your heart.

[wife]   This really hit us right between the eyes. We didn't see it coming – he got sick so fast. So just dealing with that whole knowing that the future is so uncertain. . .

[mother]   When he first announced this had happened to him, I thought he was talking about somebody else. . . . This is how shocking it was.

[wife]   When you have a week like this, it's hard because you went from a really good place to an unknown place, which is the worst. Once you know what you're dealing with, it's crappy, but it's something tangible that you know what you're dealing with. When you have these unknowns I think it makes it worse, and it's frustrating.

[wife]   He was feeling so wonderfully that we are very surprised he has cancer. He always looked well, ate well, and there was really nothing. As I say, we were stunned because physically, mentally, everything was perfect.

Participants described the experience of hearing the diagnosis as "life-changing." They said they felt forcibly shoved into a new world in which they were unfamiliar with the language and customs, and did not have a vision of how they would survive.

[friend]   When you're in there you feel isolated. You feel, the world is different, you know there are many people in your situation, but you're kind of in your own sphere.

[husband]   I have been here and I see young people and it is devastating. It really is. It is a devastating disease.

[husband]   I remember the day we went to see the doctor, the oncologist, after the lung biopsy. . . . I was really shaking. . . . I was like a basket case. I was in worse shape than she was . . . the uncertainty, the shock, the fear of losing someone you have loved for so long, who is – [crying] so much of your life.

They yearned for their old lives prior to the diagnosis.

[daughter]   It's like one of those things – you wish you could wave a magic wand and go back in time.

[wife]   Our whole life is being changed from before as we knew it. It may continue to change. . . . What the plan is?. . . . Where's the old life?

Frequently, the caregivers spoke of the diagnosis as a pivotal point in time – there was life before the diagnosis, the shock of the diagnosis, followed by the new era of fear and uncertainty. They reported being worried about having to deal with so many unknown factors simultaneously.

[domestic partner]   I haven't been sleeping well, because I just lay there and things just run over and over and over in my head. A lot of times I find myself worrying about so much stuff. If we have a huge schedule coming up for the week, a lot of doctors' visits, a lot of tests . . . just thinking about everything gets me tired! I start feeling tired before I've even started doing everything!

[wife]   Well, you know it has totally changed our life. Well – [crying] we don't know what's ahead.

[daughter]   . . . I think if I sit down and think about all the bills and all the mortgage due, this one has to go here tomorrow, and [patient] has to go to the doctor, and I have two appointments scheduled at the same time, oh my God, I have to go for bloodwork because Pop had a CAT scan yesterday, and now I need to check his creatinine level, you know, and all his medications. Dinner. Breakfast, lunch, dinner. . . . Who is taking what pill?

With the pervasive influence of shock, fear, and uncertainty, it was extremely difficult for caregivers to ascribe meaning to their family member's illness. A few caregivers ascribed negative meaning, saying the cancer was punishment from God for their family member's past behaviors (Williams, Dixon, Feinn, & McCorkle, 2015). Some caregivers expressed bitterness and anger toward their ill family member.

[wife]   Life was so good. And, you know, you're going from that perspective of . . . Okay, we can start coasting a little bit and enjoying life. And, then a week later we had the rug pulled out from underneath us. It just seemed so unfair – [crying] It's not supposed to work that way, and I was angry. I was real angry. First, I was angry at him [the patient]. I was angry at God . . . and I was feeling sorry for myself . . . like why me? – that kind of feeling sorry.

[husband]   So, when my wife was first diagnosed . . . we both said this would be a test of our faith because . . . it was God who gave her that.

[husband]   We fight all the time now because . . . she takes everything the wrong way. She's very on edge. I just try to stay away from her because she's

not happy and I just leave her alone, let her sit. She sat all weekend – distant, staring into space. Part of it is because I said something to her and she took it the wrong way . . . started screaming and yelling and got mad at me. She didn't want to talk to me and I said fine.

[daughter]   So part of you feels guilty because . . . part of you is almost angry at it all, and then you're like that's not fair to be angry at him because he's the one going through it.

[wife]   I am ashamed of being angry at [patient] . . . I felt how dare I. I was ashamed that I felt that way, but I was angry with him because for so many years he smoked despite my nagging and despite my whatever, and that was why I was angry because he chose that lifestyle habit. So that's why I was angry because my thought was if you didn't smoke, you wouldn't have this right now.

[wife]   He was diagnosed with lung cancer and the family was angry because he didn't take care of himself. . . . I would come home from work and he would be sitting in the garage, and he would be smoking. I would go through the roof.

[brother]   Cancer is man's foolishness to alter some kind of substance: cigarettes, tobacco, meat or anything else to make it better and make more money from it, and it affects our bodies. God doesn't punish us, we punish ourselves.

[wife]   I think my situation is I'm angry. I'm angry with God that now it's all on me.

POST-SURGERY

The patients cared for by the family caregivers in this study tended to have extensive surgeries with physically demanding periods of convalescence. During the time immediately after surgery, the caregiver's focus often shifted to the responsibility of providing physical care. With a steep learning curve for the caregiver to acquire skills in wound care, surgical drains, and medication management, caregivers spoke about being highly task oriented and attentive to pragmatic concerns to get them through the day. It was not uncommon for caregivers to report pride in successfully executing their new skills and being of tangible assistance to their ill family member.

[husband]   . . . I found resources within me to help my wife through the emotional trauma of this . . . to be a good person beyond I suppose what I had been in life. It was really surprising and I suppose in a way gratifying that I had those resources, that I could rise to the occasion and provide her with the help that she needed and to do so in a – surprisingly for myself – accepting fashion.

[wife]   Well, it's interesting. I think if you had asked me five months ago to describe what a day would be like and if I was able to do it, I would have said, "Absolutely not. I'm not going to be strong enough to do this." Somehow, I have found the strength, and I do consider it an honor to take care of him. I had to learn how to give injections and monitor his

blood, give fifty different pills and deal with the fact that he is extremely depressed.

[husband]   I find myself growing in some respects because of it. I find myself doing more, being . . . more patient with other people. . . . I find myself a little patient because I'm dedicating – you know, seeing if she's okay, seeing that she's not cold, if there is more I can do. . . . So I have improved in some respects. . . . I seem to be a bit more grounded now. I don't know if that's true, but it feels true.

[wife]   After surgery you're supposed to come home and heal, but instead he kept going in and out and coming home with TPN and drains, and all kinds of fun stuff at home. So we have a little infirmary in the dining room [laughs].

[wife]   Emotionally it has been very hard. The emotional aspects are as hard as the physical aspects. I have to shower him, get him to the bathroom, do all that, but that's not as hard as maybe the down times when he's sleeping twenty-two hours a day, and I don't leave him.

[daughter]   It's hard. It's by far the hardest thing I've ever done, and I know that it's going to get harder. It is brutal, but I'm very honored and privileged to be able to do it. I feel very lucky.

As for meaning making – many caregivers spoke about the cancer as if it were a teacher. The cancer brought their family together and taught them to see the importance of their relationships and to enjoy the little things in life.

[daughter]   Being a caregiver is a great gift, especially because it's my mom that has been diagnosed with cancer. . . . It's an unfortunate thing but it's a way to celebrate life knowing at least it's not a car accident, she's gone, we didn't have time. . . . So it's wonderful to spend the one-on-one time. I think it's a great gift we have been given.

[friend]   I think that in times like this, it brings people closer together because it's like you're going through it with them – although not the actual pain and discomfort, but you feel their pain oftentimes. And then you start to share things that you normally wouldn't say because you're more vulnerable, that person is more vulnerable so they're opening up more about how they're feeling. We tend to mask how we're feeling and stuff, but when it's a serious thing like this you tend to be more open so I find that to be a very positive thing.

[son]   Cancer was not an easy thing to take from the beginning. In our case, in terms of family, it has pulled us together a little bit, a lot more. . . . I guess when the whole thing started, everybody just . . . you know, you have a lot more phone calls. You have a lot more visits. You have a lot more – "How are you feeling?" All of a sudden someone will show up with groceries like fruits and anything like that just to kind of say, "Here I am." It's kind of nice to have people looking over your back. Just kind of showing up every once and a while out of the blue. You know it's

because he has cancer, but they don't want to make it seem like that, but they do show up. I guess that's a good side to it. Something that came out of it. Something positive.

[daughter] We actually look at this as a gift, because not everybody has a chance to reflect on their life before they die. When you're given this kind of diagnosis, I almost think that it makes you look at things differently. . . . I actually think it could be a gift to each of us in a different way. It's awful. It's not something that anybody wants. . . . It is definitely a life-changing experience, but you know it's been two months. I feel like where we are today versus where we were two months ago is worlds apart.

[wife] It makes you stop running around and think about things and putting things in order and prioritize what's important.

[husband] I believe – and also this experience I hope she would never get ill – but it put our family all together. It bonded everybody together, especially with the kids and me and yeah. . . . It opens your eyes to what is more important in life. You know, instead of running, she was running the same way like I did, you know, working, making sure there is a career over there, positions, money and everything, and one day she said screw it, I don't need this stuff. You know, health is more important.

CHEMOTHERAPY

When their family members started chemotherapy and experienced untoward side effects like nausea, vomiting, insomnia, agitation, fatigue, infections, and bowel changes, the caregivers frequently expressed weariness. In some cases, the family caregivers experienced overwhelming despair that colored any meaning they might have been able to derive from their experience.

[cousin] I think that given the feeling of being pulled in so many different directions where you finally realize that I am being stretched beyond belief here . . . that you just need to sit back and. . . . I've honestly had moments like that where I thought – I just can't do this!

[daughter] It is my responsibility to be there for her now, but it has become more of a chore and not a choice.

[wife] He was very sick, he never realized how sick he was. I went to church and I said [to God], "I can't do this by myself anymore." Next I said, "You've got to do it, I can't do it!"

[daughter] It has become extremely overwhelming, and it has become who I am. That is who I am now. I am my mother's caretaker and I'm kind of losing myself, and as much as I want to help her there are days where I don't. I really don't, and I resent it.

To these caregivers, it seemed as if they were catapulting from one crisis to the next. They felt like they did not have time to catch their breath or adjust to the new circumstances before another challenge appeared. Meaning was elusive for many. A few caregivers said the cancer (or God) was testing their mettle and they felt determined to show they could persevere. Others felt the cancer was a crucible meant to humble them (or their ill family member) so that they could start life anew.

[wife]   I'm sleep deprived. . . . I was up at five today and I've got a son I have to worry about . . . he's home alone . . . so there's all of that . . . and the dogs and wondering if we have orange juice. So, all of the minutia and then worrying about [patient] . . . and he's starting this new drug that we just signed forms agreeing to our awareness of the twenty different side effects . . . the future is just so mysterious now.

[daughter]   Probably because I find that as the days go on with dealing with my mom's illness and my son's illness, I find it's getting harder and harder to cope with it and to understand why it's happening to both the people that I care for. . . . You just take it one day at a time . . . just overall I'm feeling angry.

[brother]   If God gives you a thing to do, you can't escape it. It's nothing great that you're doing. It's just like, okay, for all you've done, now you have to go out and carry this cross for me. Sometimes it gets emotional when I think about it [crying].

[son]   I started growing up a lot more. I started taking on responsibilities like around the house. . . . I have been trying to step it up more. It's kind of taught me a lot of responsibility. She's trying to teach me now as much as she can . . . while we still have time.

PASSAGE OF TIME

Often family caregivers spoke about time as if it were a sentient being capable of speeding up and slowing down at will. When their patient had intractable physical or emotional pain, time passed excruciatingly slowly. Similarly, when they were waiting for laboratory results or scans to confirm treatment effectiveness – time again seemed to be sluggish.

[domestic partner]   Part of the thing right now is that he's in a lot of pain, and that's why I always feel like I have to be near him because if he wants anything – it's hard for him to get up and down . . . I think once his pain eases a little bit. . . . I think I'll feel more free to take a little time back for myself. Right now, I feel like I have to be there all the time.

[wife]   I think on days when [patient] is feeling pain, or on days when he feels like he's not making any progress . . . it's moments like that, that make you think, "This day is never going to end. I don't think I'm going to make it through this day."

[wife]   We just have to wait. Waiting is a big part of everything. We're always waiting for something.

On the days when they found reprieve from disease and spent time enjoying family and friends, when they felt gratitude, love, and awakening to the preciousness of life and each other – then they reported delight in the suspension of time. The following is a longer quote from a caregiver who is also father to two young children. This caregiver is reflecting on how his experience of the passage of time and waiting for biomarker results has changed during the three-year duration of his wife's illness.

[husband]   Actually right now, it's been very interesting for the last three years, and I believe it changed my life. Before we used to sit and wait . . . okay the test in three months, what is going to happen? You know, if it is bad results or good results, usually you don't ever talk about the good results. You always think about the worst that can happen, and then my mentality completely changed. Like I will not think about this test until the day comes. You know something, the test was done two weeks ago, we are going to get the results, and *then* we are going to think about it. Right now – enjoy life, your life, you have the kids, house, everything! You know, you're healthy at this moment. What is going to happen in two weeks? . . . You know I can get ill in two weeks. Nobody knows. Nobody knows. Nobody knows. To just sit and think what is going to happen in the future, I don't think it's worth it. I don't think it's worth it anymore. You just take it day by day, and get the best of it. Take the best of that day. Enjoy your life because you never know what's going to happen. You know it is a lot, millions of innocent people dying all over the world and we are still alive, we can deal with this situation, but just try not to think what is going to happen in the week or two weeks when you see the doctor. Yeah, it's been tough. That's why I said we just continue with whatever we need to do, and give it every six months, three months off, you know we can enjoy life, go on vacations like nothing happened. If it comes back, we deal with that situation when it comes. When the situation comes back and we need to go back to the doctors, then deal with the situation with whatever cancer comes back, then that is what we have got to do. But we need to wait the time. I believe we need to wait the time.

SUMMARY: CANCER FAMILY CAREGIVER INTERVIEWS

The cancer family caregivers quoted earlier speak with candor about the intimate and challenging experience of caring for someone with a life-altering illness. Their words paint a vivid picture of the arduous journey patients and their families undertake from time of diagnosis through post-surgical care and chemotherapy. The interweave of time, mind, and body is explicit when they express their shock, anger, and feelings of being overwhelmed concurrent with high physical and psychological burden of disease; as well as when they express hope, gratitude, love, and transformational growth with the passage of time and the ability to find meaning in the experience. In the next section, Fusion of Time, Mind, and Body: Revisited, I continue discussing the cancer family caregivers' experiences.

FUSION OF TIME, MIND, AND BODY: REVISITED

An expanse of time offers us the opportunity to see patterns amid chaos and acclimate to new and scary situations. However, rarely in healthcare do patients get to decide the timing of events and claim the expanse of time that they need. This is one way objective time seems to be a malevolent presence, as patients and health professionals conform to schedules structured for mass production not meaning making – or perhaps, not even adequate healthcare. Is it possible to experience subjectively the dilation of time needed to derive meaning from illness? Philosophy, cognitive science, and some of the cancer family caregivers who described their experiences earlier indicate the answer is yes. Let's explore this question more fully by revisiting the fusion of time, mind, and body.

The connection between bodily experiences and consciousness are abundant in the family caregiver quotes posted above. Whether the family caregiver personally experienced physical and/or psychic pain or experienced pain vicariously through the patient, appears to be inconsequential. In both instances, illness burden expressed by the body affected the family caregiver's ability to derive meaning from their situation. You may have noticed that when the caregivers conveyed psychic pain (e.g., fear, uncertainty, anger), they were either unable to find meaning in the experience or they found negative meaning (e.g., punishment from God). When the caregivers had specific tasks to do, typically in the post-surgical phase, they felt good about themselves and described positive effects on their family from the cancer experience (e.g., bringing family together, reprioritizing their lives). Unfortunately, when the tasks became too numerous or too demanding, the caregivers quickly became overwhelmed, and the illness experience was devoid of meaning. Especially in the presence of pain, consciousness is muted and one's sense of time is ablated. The caregiver interviews demonstrate the tenuous balance among temporality, consciousness, and corporeality.

THE HEALTH PROFESSIONAL

While exploring the influence of time on meaning, I have primarily highlighted the experience of the patient and family. Let's now consider what health professionals might extrapolate from this discussion. Like patients and family members, we *make time* for the patient encounter, *spend time* developing the therapeutic relationship, and wait – sometimes waiting for laboratory and imaging studies to determine the diagnosis, sometimes waiting for a disease to declare itself, sometimes waiting for treatment effects, and all the while working with uncertainty. Working with uncertainty can be a major hurdle for health professionals, and if that hurdle is not cleared can lead to high stress, professional burnout, and other consequences. I discuss uncertainty in chapter 5 Resilience and Burnout, and explore the topic of uncertainty in detail in chapter 8 Uncertainty and Shared Decision Making.

As health professionals, we may have periods when it is challenging to find meaning in our work, especially when we are depleted physically and emotionally (see chapter 4 Bearing Witness to Suffering and chapter 5 Resilience and Burnout). Whether we are depleted from the demands of providing healthcare or our personal desolation, it is important to recall the dynamic relationship among temporality, consciousness, and corporeality. We need periodically to give ourselves time to refresh our minds and bodies, and reflect on our personal and professional experiences. When our reflection uses the construct and power of story to equilibrate mind and body, we have the potential to discover meaning. Our stories are not only an expression of our lived experience, which by definition is a manifestation of our past, but our stories are also a beacon for how we live in the present and certainly inform our decisions for the future. The human experience, be it your relationship with a lover, your health professional education, normal aging, or illness, is ever changing. The human experience essentially decrees that meaning will change over time.

INVITATION TO ATTEND TO THE INFLUENCE OF TIME IN YOUR LIFE

I invite you to pay attention in your own life to how your thoughts and feelings about major events, and the meaning you attribute to them, change under the influence of time. One simple way to do this is to keep a journal. If you are too busy to journal regularly, I encourage you to at least jot notes about your thoughts and feelings about upcoming or present moment events that you perceive as life changing. Some examples of life-changing events are: starting health professional school, having one of your patients die, attending a birth, having a family member or friend die, getting married, getting divorced, becoming a parent, experiencing an empty nest, sustaining a debilitating injury, being diagnosed with a chronic disease. Once you have written your notes, mark your calendar for a time in the future to read what you have written. It can be startling to see how our perceptions change over time. When our perceptions do *not* change over time, it is valuable to reflect on why they have endured.

SERIAL WRITING PROMPTS AND REFLECTION

For many years, I have invited my students (physician assistant, nursing, and medical) to write down their thoughts and feelings at the beginning of their human anatomy dissection course. The students then seal their writing in envelopes and the envelopes are stored securely until the end of anatomy. As the anatomy course draws to a close, I again invite the students to write about their experience of human anatomy dissection, this time reflecting on how their experience changed from the beginning of the course and how they anticipate it might change in the future. The students then compare their writing from the beginning of human anatomy dissection to their writing composed at the conclusion of dissection. Although the second writing prompt specifically asks the students to consider change in their experience over time, a few students every year are not able to identify change. As I remind the students, not experiencing change is interesting too. It is always worthwhile to reflect on what contributes to intransigence in our lives.

CLOSING

We have barely grazed the surface of the topic of time and the considerable influence it has on us. In this chapter, we used conceptual work in philosophy and cognitive science to provide a foundation for our discussion of time. We explored the influence of time on patients', family members', and health professionals' experiences of illness, and looked at how meaning changes over time, especially with changes in body and mind. We read excerpts from individual interviews with cancer family caregivers, who described their experiences at the time of their ill family member's diagnosis, and when caring for their ill family member after surgery and during chemotherapy. The family caregivers' stories demonstrated the profound persuasion temporality, consciousness, and corporeality have on each other, and collectively have on one's ability to derive meaning from illness.

I close this chapter with learning objectives and reading and writing activities so the reader may have personal engagement with the influence of time on meaning.

ACTIVITIES

LEARNING OBJECTIVES

Learners will

1   discuss the influence of time on the meaning individuals may ascribe to significant life events, including illness;
2   reflect on their early personal experience with the influence of time on meaning.

SHORT STORY AND DISCUSSION

First, read the short story, *Quill*, by Tony Earley (2006). As you read, note words or passages that appeal to you, repel you, resonate with you, startle you, or in some way catch your attention. Drawing on material presented in chapter 7, reflect on the influence of time on the meaning the characters in the short story ascribe to events both past and present.

SMALL GROUP DISCUSSION

Learners are invited to discuss their experience with the short story. Whenever possible, learners should refer to specific passages in the short story. In particular, learners should aim to comment on the influence of time on meaning. Faculty facilitators may choose to ask someone to read aloud a passage from the story that captured their attention. Reading aloud makes the text a presence in the room and helps everyone focus. If at all possible, allow the conversation about the text to evolve organically, directed by the learners' curiosity.

NOTE: **Appendix A** has general guidelines for facilitating a health humanities seminar. **Appendix B** has instruction and discussion prompts specific to this activity for faculty facilitators to use if your learners are not able to initiate a robust discussion.

WRITING AND SHARING

The second activity is for the learner to write to a prompt that directly links the chapter content and the short story. Here is a suggested writing prompt:

> Write about an experience that has been influenced by time. Feel free to write fiction.

Faculty facilitators can invite the learners to share what they have written with the group. Learners should never be required to share their writings.

REFERENCE LIST

Crystal, D. (2002). Talking about time. In K. Ridderbos (Ed.), *Time* (pp. 105–125). New York: Cambridge University Press.

Droit-Volet, S., & Gil, S. (2009). The time-emotion paradox. *Philosophical Transactions of the Royal Society B, 364*(1525), 1943–1954.

Eagleman, D. M. (2008). Human time perception and its illusions. *Current Opinion in Neurobiology, 18*(2), 131–136.

Earley, T. (2006). Quill. In J. Thomas & R. Shapard (Eds.), *Flash fiction forward* (pp. 168–170). New York: W. W. Norton & Company.

Halifax, J. (2008). *Being with dying: Cultivating compassion and fearlessness in the presence of death*. Boston, MA: Shambala.

International Society for the Study of Time. (n.d.). *New ISST tri-fold flyer*. Author. Retrieved from www.studyoftime.org/ISST-trifold-US.pdf

Kleinman, A., Eisenberg, L., & Good, B. (1978). Culture, illness, and care: Clinical lessons from anthropologic and cross-cultural research. *Annals of Internal Medicine, 88*, 251–258.

Lorde, A. (1997). *The cancer journals* (special ed.). San Francisco, CA: Aunt Lute Books.

Morris, D. B. (2010). Intractable pain and the perception of time: Every patient is an anecdote. In C. Stannard, E. Kalso, & J. Ballantyne (Eds.), *Evidence-based chronic pain management* (pp. 52–64). Oxford: Wiley-Blackwell.

St. Augustine. (2014). *The confessions of St. Augustine*. Translated by A. Outler. Leadership U Cyber Library. Retrieved from www.leaderu.com/cyber/books/augconfessions/bk11.html

Thomas, S. P., & Johnson, M. (2000). A phenomenologic study of chronic pain. *Western Journal of Nursing Research, 22*, 683–705.

van Wassenhove, V., Wittman, M., Craig, A. D., & Paulus, M. P. (2011). Psychological and neural mechanisms of subjective time dilation. *Frontiers in Neuroscience, 5*(56). doi:10.3389/fnins.2011.0056

Weinert, F. (2013). *The march of time: Evolving conceptions of time in the light of scientific discoveries*. Berlin and Heidelberg, DE: Springer Verlag.

Williams, A. L., & Bakitas, M. (2012). Cancer family caregivers: A new direction for interventions. *Journal of Palliative Medicine, 15*(7), 775–783.

Williams, A. L., Dixon, J., Feinn, R., & McCorkle, R. (2015). Cancer family caregiver depression: Are religion-related variables important? *Psycho-Oncology, 24*, 825–831.

Wittman, M. (2016). *Felt time: The psychology of how we perceive time*. Translated by E. Butler. Cambridge, MA and London: MIT Press.

8 UNCERTAINTY AND DECISION MAKING

INTEGRATION NOTE
....

This chapter integrates with study of health communication, cross-cultural care, diagnostic reasoning, and diagnostic probability. The learner activities at the end of the chapter complement instruction related to gastrointestinal diseases.

INTRODUCTION

Uncertainty permeates many aspects of healthcare delivery. We like to think that biomedical science drives clinical practice and thus lends us the certitude of scientific inquiry. In reality, each patient is unique, so consequently many scientific facts do not apply to individual cases. As described in the Australian report, *Complexity and Healthcare: Health Practitioner Workforce, Services, Roles, Skills and Training to Respond to Patients with Complex Needs*, medical complexity includes co-morbid conditions and treatments, and situational complexity arises from the patient's personal, social, economic, behavioral, and cultural factors (Kuipers et al., 2011). The coupling of medical complexity and situational complexity yields multiple interrelated variables and few, if any, resources that help health professionals unambiguously address clinical care.

Uncertainty in healthcare becomes even more pronounced when we consider the issue of publication bias. Publication bias means that studies with negative results are rarely distributed in high profile biomedical journals, and intervention adverse effects, especially from pharmaceuticals, are grossly underreported (Golder, Loke, Wright, & Norman, 2016). Subsequently, health professionals are left to rely on a tainted evidence base (Unnikrishnana, 2017). Even when we have confidence in our clinical acumen as health professionals, we still must work with the uncertain quality of the biomedical evidence pool. Health professionals and patients are required routinely to make decisions in uncertain circumstances.

In this chapter, I examine the theoretical underpinnings of uncertainty. I describe the characteristics of complex adaptive systems and explore how health and healthcare express those characteristics. I then examine the literature that describes the effect uncertainty has on health professionals and patients. The uncertainty of the healthcare system is an important and vast topic, especially in the United States where legislation about access to and coverage of healthcare services is in flux (Starr, 2013). Healthcare system uncertainty is beyond the scope of this chapter and will not be covered here. Rather, my focus is on health professionals and patients who tolerate and manage uncertainty throughout the illness experience, and especially while making serious treatment decisions. Often the patient's family must also tolerate and manage uncertainty. Chapter 7 Influence of Time on Meaning, Influence of Time on Our Understanding of Illness section, presents qualitative data from cancer family caregivers about their experience with uncertainty, therefore I will not revisit the family experience here. Later in the chapter, I share some interventions to improve health professionals' tolerance for uncertainty and strengthen one's ability to work with uncertainty in healthcare. I highlight key features involved in making a decision, with a focus on decisions made in the context of medical uncertainty. Finally, I present ideas about how shared decision making is influenced by the health professional–patient relationship, and how that in turn influences health outcomes. I close the chapter with activities that provide opportunity for experiential learning related to uncertainty and decision making.

UNCERTAINTY

DEFINITION: SOURCE, ISSUE, AND LOCUS

Let's begin our discussion of uncertainty by establishing a working definition. In the article, "Varieties of Uncertainty in Health Care: A Conceptual Taxonomy," authors Han, Klein, and Arora (2011) define uncertainty as "the subjective perception of ignorance" (p. 830). In other words, uncertainty is the internal state of mind or belief that one has insufficient knowledge for a given situation. The germinal work of Lipshitz and Strauss (1997) deconstructs uncertainty based on *source* and *issue*. Uncertainty source derives from incomplete information, inadequate understanding of the information, or the inability to differentiate between seemingly equal alternatives. Uncertainty issue refers to the particular outcomes, situations, or roles that are imposed by deciding on one of the alternatives.

Han et al. (2011) propose an uncertainty conceptual framework which further defines source and issue dimensions, and adds the dimension of *locus*. They define source dimension not simply as ambiguity among alternatives, but also include probabilistic unreliability and acknowledgement that complex situations (like illness and healthcare) involve multiple variables that decrease the likelihood that reliable information exists. The issue dimension is further categorized as scientific, practical, and personal. In terms of healthcare, scientific uncertainties relate to diagnosis, prognosis, and treatment recommendations. Practical uncertainties range from a patient's concern about the quality and competency of his or her healthcare worker to transportation issues and costs to access care. Personal uncertainty encompasses the effects of illness on one's goals, relationships, and sense of meaning in life. Locus, the new dimension of uncertainty presented in the Han et al. (2011) framework, refers to where (or rather, in whom) the uncertainty exists. Since uncertainty is a subjective perception, it can manifest in the mind of the health professional, the patient, or both. As we will discuss in the Decision Making section that follows, regardless of in whom the uncertainty originates, it ideally becomes a shared experience between the health professional and patient, with each contributing to its mitigation. To summarize, uncertainty is "the subjective perception of ignorance." It is comprised of three dimensions (source, issue, and locus) which characterize the type and origin of the uncertainty (Han et al., 2011).

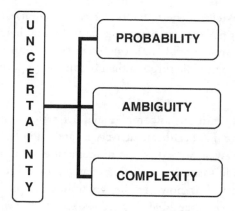

Figure 8.1 Relationships among uncertainty, probability, ambiguity, and complexity.
Adapted from Hillen et al., 2017. Figure 3. Sources of Uncertainty. *Social Science & Medicine*,
180, 72.

As this chapter continues, I talk about uncertainty, ambiguity, and complexity. Figure 8.1
shows the relationships among these constructs. Uncertainty is the umbrella construct
that is comprised of probability (e.g., inherent unpredictability, stochastic variability),
ambiguity (e.g., conflicting, imprecise, missing information), and complexity (e.g.,
multiple causal factors) (Hillen, Cutheil, Strout, Smets, & Han, 2017).

COMPLEX ADAPTIVE SYSTEMS: HEALTH AND HEALTHCARE

Complexity science emerged in response to the recognition that complex adaptive
systems require non-linear functioning. In other words, there are no simple solutions to
complex problems. Key characteristics of complex adaptive systems, including health and
healthcare, are that the systems: consist of interactive components; have multi-level and
multi-directional interactions among the components; are defined by the relationships
among the components; cannot be reduced to specific components; are dynamic and
evolving (Sturmberg & Martin, 2013).

Let's look briefly at how the characteristics of complex adaptive systems are expressed in
health and healthcare. Physiologic health is achieved through intricate, dynamic interplay
among organ systems and the environment. A modest change in function of one organ
system leads to compensation among the other organ systems. Similarly, minor variations
in the environment can have devastating effects on individual organ systems and the body
as a whole. The body is in a continuous state of recalibration to internal and external
forces, always seeking equilibrium. Healthcare is also a complex adaptive system in that it
is a delicate interaction between patient variables, healthcare worker variables, and access
variables. A defect or deficit in any one of the variables affects the entire system. For
example, if the nurse practitioner is a brilliant diagnostician who correctly identifies her
patient's disease and gives her patient a prescription for the optimal medication to treat his
malady, the patient still may not recover. The countervailing variables include, among a
host of others, the patient's co-morbidities, the patient's willingness and ability to adhere
to the treatment regimen, drug-drug interactions, and drug-nutrition interactions (See

chapter 2 Patient as Storyteller, Determinants of Health section). Iona Heath, MD (2013, p. 19), writing about her patient care experience says, "Seeing this situation as a complex adaptive system is much more useful . . . because sensitivity, intuition, commitment and a pragmatic preparedness to muddle through then become as important as a sound grasp of biomedical knowledge."

Appreciating health and healthcare as complex adaptive systems allows health professionals to recognize that healthcare delivery is rarely simple, and guard against the tendency to accept easy answers that lead to premature cessation of our inquiries. Diagnostic algorithms and treatment guidelines may put us in intellectual proximity to an individual patient's concerns, however, they are unlikely to predict outcomes for *that* patient. A perspective piece in the *New England Journal of Medicine* by Simpkin and Schwartzstein (2016) suggests that health professionals who practice clinical medicine with certainty are likely deluded by their own hidden assumptions and unconscious biases. When health professionals are oriented toward complexity, we develop the capacity to view intractable clinical encounters with optimism, rather than being defeated by the sheer magnitude of unpredictability, variability, and uncertainty that is inherent in most, if not all, patient care.

THE CHALLENGE OF UNCERTAINTY FOR HEALTH PROFESSIONALS AND PATIENTS

Columbia University professor, physician, and author, Siddhartha Mukherjee, MD (2015, p. 6), writes in his book, *The Laws of Medicine: Field Notes from an Uncertain Science*,

> I had never expected medicine to be such a lawless, uncertain world. . . .
> The profusion of facts obscured a deeper and more significant problem: the reconciliation between knowledge (certain, fixed, perfect, concrete) and clinical wisdom (uncertain, fluid, imperfect, abstract).

Uncertainty is an inherent component of illness for health professionals and patients. For an otherwise healthy person who presents with a common disorder that responds quickly to therapy, uncertainty is negligible and resolves readily. An example of the quick resolution of uncertainty might be a previously healthy 25-year-old man who presents with an itchy, red rash on his hands that appeared one day after he started using new dish soap. The patient knows the offending agent that caused his rash (the dish soap) and he is easily able to remove the agent from his environment. The health professional is able to hasten the patient's recovery by giving him a topical steroid sample at no cost. Patient and health professional leave the encounter satisfied and confident that the diagnosis of contact dermatitis is accurate and the treatment will be safe and effective.

As medical and situational complexity increase, uncertainty becomes a greater challenge and more ominous threat. Additionally, when confronted with high medical and situational complexity, we are less able to rely on the body of scientific evidence to predict our patients' outcomes. For example, there is scientific evidence to support the use of statin drugs to treat hypercholesterolemia and reduce the relative risk of myocardial infarction. However, much of that scientific evidence is derived from studies of white men (Truong, Murphy, McCabe, Armani, & Cannon, 2011). At present, there is no scientific evidence that tells us how statin drugs will affect an obese, 40-year-old, menstruating woman who concomitantly takes synthetic thyroid for Hashimoto's thyroiditis, glucophage for pre-diabetes, receives three chemotherapy drugs for non-small cell carcinoma of the lung, and consumes unlabeled herbal teas and oils sent from relatives. Beyond the paucity of knowledge about how drugs affect people who are not white men and how drugs interact with other chemicals, we also do not know how drugs interact with psychosocial factors such as patient employment, housing, family dynamics, and religious practices (Kuipers et al., 2011).

A 2011 discussion paper presented by members of the European Association for Quality in General Practice/Family Medicine (2011, p. 177) states,

> There are many consultations where there are no straight answers, no clear diagnosis and no obvious treatment, where guidelines and decision-making protocols do not lead to a satisfactory outcome. In this situation, at one extreme the doctor who believes in their own infallibility when faced with diagnostic decisions can be a source of danger, as can the doctor at the other extreme who struggles with indecision on a daily basis.

As health professionals, we have to find the balance between stridency and hesitancy, and learn to work effectively with uncertainty. Later in this chapter, I present interventions that may help us achieve that balance (see Interventions to Tolerate Uncertainty).

PSYCHOLOGY OF UNCERTAINTY

What effect does working with uncertainty have on health professionals? The short answer is – it depends on the person. We each have our own threshold for tolerating uncertainty and ambiguity that is set by our confidence level and sense of control (Penrod, 2007). Additional moderators of our individual tolerance for uncertainty include sociocultural factors, personal characteristics, and the environment in which we are experiencing the uncertainty (Hillen et al., 2017). Once we cross our personal threshold we begin to feel varying degrees of cognitive, emotional, and behavioral discomfort, which may motivate us to see opportunity, be curious, and seek creative solutions, or incite us to feel vulnerable, be fearful, and aim to avoid the situation (Schneider et al., 2010).

HEALTH PROFESSIONAL BURDEN

Several reports describe difficulties that health professionals endure from working with uncertainty, namely high stress, burnout, increased consultations, and excessive diagnostic study orders. Unfortunately, there are few studies that use data to document the burden from uncertainty. I highlight one recent quantitative study of physicians and two qualitative studies of nurses.

A 2017 study of Italian physicians assessed intolerance for uncertainty and ambiguity, and the need for cognitive closure as predictors of perceived stress (Iannelo, Mottini,

Tirelli, Riva, & Antonietti, 2017). The sample (N = 212) included men and women with varying years of practice (< 10 years, 10–20 years, > 20 years) who worked in 18 different specialties. There were no significant differences between genders, years of practice categories, or specialties on any of the self-report questionnaires (perceived stress, tolerance for ambiguity, stress from uncertainty, preference for order, preference for predictability, decisiveness, discomfort with ambiguity, and closed-mindedness). Multivariate regression modeling showed that after controlling for gender and practice specialty, four variables predicted physicians with elevated perceived work-related stress: low tolerance for ambiguity, high stress from uncertainty, low decisiveness, and less than 10 years of practice. The strongest predictor of work-related stress was an elevated score on the questionnaire assessing stress from uncertainty.

Researchers conducted in-depth semi-structured interviews with intensive care unit nurses (N = 14) at two Canadian academic medical centers. The goal of the study was to develop a grounded theory to explain the experience of uncertainty among nurses in clinical practice (Cranley, Doran, Tourangeau, Kushniruk, & Nagle, 2012). Participants described three clinical situations that contributed to their feelings of uncertainty: 1) "feeling caught off-guard" by a disease with which they had little professional experience or a patient who was physiologically unstable; 2) "encountering unfamiliar or unique orders"; and 3) "navigating the ethical gray areas of practice" such as when there are differing treatment goals among the physicians, nurses, and patient, or when there is no obvious correct course of care (p. 152). Several participants reported emotional responses to uncertain clinical situations, such as feeling uncomfortable, frustrated, and emotionally drained. Some nurses reported physiologic stress responses and anxiety. While a few nurses described being overwhelmed, others said the uncertainty heightened their focus and conscientiousness.

Using qualitative descriptive methodology, researchers conducted semi-structured interviews with female nurses who worked on medical and surgical wards at an academic medical center in Iran (N = 18) (Vaismoradi, Salsali, & Ahmadi, 2011). Content analysis of the transcribed interviews revealed three main themes: 1) "unclear domain of practice"; 2) "compatibility with uncertainty"; and 3) "psychological reactions to uncertainty" (p. 994). When the nurses encountered uncertain clinical situations they described feeling "frustration, anger, agitation and fear" (p. 996).

The three studies just described include physicians and nurses practicing in Italy, Canada, and Iran. While the studies are limited by their small samples, it is interesting to see the degree of overlap among the study populations as they report on their experiences of uncertainty in clinical care. Before we discuss effective ways of working with uncertainty, let's look at uncertainty with the illness experience from the patient's perspective.

PATIENT BURDEN
Professor Merle Mishel, PhD, RN, FAAN conducted the foundational work on patients' experience of uncertainty during illness. In the 1980s, Professor Mishel (1981, 1988) developed the Theory of Uncertainty in Illness, as well as the psychometrically sound

measurement tool, Uncertainty in Illness Scale. Her original theory of uncertainty derives from the perspectives of patients with acute diagnoses. Subsequently, Professor Mishel (1991) re-conceptualized the theory to apply to patients with chronic disease who must live with ongoing uncertainty. Professor Mishel (1991, p. 256) defines uncertainty as "the inability to determine the meaning of illness-related events occurring when the decision maker is unable to assign definite value to objects or events or is unable to predict outcomes accurately." The purpose of the theory is to explicate how patients cognitively process the fact that they have an illness, manage their illness-related activities (e.g., wound care, medication management, dietary modifications, mobility alterations, changes in independence), and ascribe meaning to their illness. Professor Mishel (1983) proposes four domains for patient uncertainty in illness: 1) ambiguity concerning the meaning of symptoms; 2) complexity regarding the effect of treatment upon symptoms; 3) deficient information concerning diagnosis; and 4) unpredictability concerning outcome.

HEALTH PROFESSIONAL–PATIENT UNCERTAINTY INTERACTION

As you can see from the previous two sections, the concurrence between patient and health professional perspectives on uncertainty is high. From both the patient's and the health professional's viewpoint, the presence of unpredictability and information deficit in complex clinical scenarios is challenging. This raises the question – is there an interdependent relationship between health professionals' and patients' experiences of uncertainty? Apparently, this is a relatively unexplored query. Portnoy, Han, Ferrer, Klein, and Clauser (2013) "examined how physicians' perceptions of their patients' tolerance of uncertainty, in addition to physician and practice characteristics, are related to attitudes toward disclosing information and involving patients in decisions about medical interventions characterized by scientific uncertainty" (p. 363). Researchers used self-report surveys from primary care physicians (N = 1500) to determine their preferred communication pattern with patients (full disclosure, patient autonomy, paternalism, withholding intervention), and their perceptions of patients' ambiguity aversion. Although there was some variability by specialty, years in practice, gender, and race, results showed that, generally speaking, physicians perceive that a large percentage of their patients will have negative reactions (i.e., ambiguity aversion) if they disclose scientific uncertainty. Furthermore, the physicians' perceptions of their patients' negative reactions had bearing on their communication patterns. Physician perception of patient ambiguity aversion significantly predicted physician reticence to communicate scientific uncertainty with patients. The study did not confirm the accuracy of the physicians' perceptions of their patients' ambiguity aversion. If the physicians' perceptions and the patients' actual aversion do not align, then the patient is effectively bereft of the physician as a knowledge resource that could potentially mollify uncertainty.

Iona Heath, MD (2013, p. 22) writes,

> The crucial conversations within health care occur between patients and clinicians, and complexity science suggests that health services should be organized to maximize and to sustain these conversations. The outcome of these conversations

is always uncertain and if an authentic interaction is achieved both parties become caught up in it and neither controls it.

Later in the chapter, I explore how components of the "crucial conversations within healthcare," which Dr. Heath prioritizes, serve patients and health professionals (see Decision Making section).

UNCERTAINTY TOLERANCE

Once we acknowledge uncertainty as intrinsic to health and healthcare, then we need to figure out how to optimize our ability to tolerate uncertainty and strengthen our ability to work with uncertainty. Let's first determine what uncertainty tolerance entails, and then look at some interventions that help us dwell with confidence in situations of clinical uncertainty.

COGNITIVE, EMOTIONAL, AND BEHAVIORAL RESPONSES

In their 2017 publication, Hillen et al. present an integrative conceptual model of uncertainty tolerance. Based on narrative review and conceptual analysis of 18 instruments that measure uncertainty and ambiguity tolerance, the authors synthesize multidisciplinary perspectives to create an organizing framework. The integrative model of uncertainty tolerance shows that when we perceive uncertainty we have cognitive, emotional, and behavioral responses, each of which can be either negative or positive. A negative cognitive response may be to perceive threat and vulnerability, or deny or doubt that a situation exists; whereas a positive cognitive response may be to perceive opportunity from the challenge and have confidence in one's ability to persevere. A negative emotional response may include worry, fear, disinterest, aversion, or despair; whereas a positive emotional response expresses calm, courage, curiosity, and hope. A negative behavioral response involves avoidance, inaction, decision deferral, or inattention; whereas a positive behavioral response embodies action, decision making, and information seeking.

How do we position ourselves to have positive cognitive, emotional, and behavioral responses to uncertainty? There is evidence that our responses are driven by our individual characteristics, such as gender, age, and personality trait. A large survey study shows uncertainty and ambiguity tolerance are highly correlated with personality trait (Lauriola, Foschi, Mosca, & Weller, 2016). Among the Big Five Inventory Personality Traits (openness to new experiences, conscientiousness, extraversion, agreeableness, and neuroticism), participants whose predominant traits were openness to new experiences and/or extraversion were more inclined to have positive responses to uncertainty and ambiguity. The understanding is that openness and extraversion traits predict active interest in a variety of situations simply for the sake of experience, thereby aligning with high tolerance for uncertainty. Individual characteristics like personality traits may not be immutable; however, they are stubbornly persistent. Does that mean that health professionals whose personality traits do not predispose them to tolerance for uncertainty are stuck being miserable while working with uncertainty in healthcare? The answer is a resounding no. Recent literature asserts that tolerance for uncertainty is a learned skill that can be cultivated. Let's take a detailed look at ways we can encourage tolerance for uncertainty in healthcare.

INTERVENTIONS TO CULTIVATE UNCERTAINTY TOLERANCE

HUMANITIES

Author and New York University professor of medicine, Danielle Ofri, MD, PhD (2017), wrote a commentary entitled, *Medical Humanities: The Rx for Uncertainty?* As the title indicates, Dr. Ofri presents a compelling case for physicians and students to spend time immersed in the humanities to learn

> a paradigm for living with ambiguity, and even for relishing it. Great works of literature, art, theater, and music specialize in ambiguity, confusion, and frailty. Unlike medicine, the humanities do not shy away from uncertainty. They revel in the depth and breadth that ambiguity affords.
>
> (p. 1657)

Dr. Ofri goes on to say,

> the medical humanities function as a photographic negative for clinical practice, bringing light to places that are normally dark. . . . They leaven the thought process to promote more nuanced thinking, something that stands to benefit both patient and doctor alike.
>
> (p. 1658)

The humanities offer us the opportunity to slow down, reflect, and consider a range of challenges and possibilities. Whether visual or literary art, philosophy, music, or social science, we are invited to pause and reflect. When we pause, it is easier to see that the division between right and wrong is often blurry, not distinct. With reflection, we allow the ethical norm of "it depends" to appear, and then we ponder those dependencies. Our perceptions expand and more aspects of life become available to us.

CREATIVE WRITING

In chapter 4 Bearing Witness to Suffering, the section Telling Our Stories discusses the salubrious effects from reflective writing. Here we will talk about creative writing. Jay Baruch, MD (2013), author and professor of emergency medicine at Warren Alpert School of Medicine at Brown University, describes the ways creative writing enriches his clinical skills. Dr. Baruch depicts the spontaneous unfolding of the clinical encounter, which more often than not includes an array of surprises that demand creative responses. He writes,

> The value and success of certain tools depend, in part, upon the talents and vision of the person using them. Any discussion of writing skills as clinical skills must also

argue for the importance of artistic habits at the bedside; this includes comfort with uncertainty and ambiguity, an embrace of mystery and conflict, a desire to challenge what is known and to push questions to uncomfortable places.

(p. 460)

How does creative writing help us with uncertainty, mystery, and conflict in healthcare? Dr. Baruch points out the nonlinearity of the creative writing process and the clinical encounter. He states,

> Writing is a humbling process for me, and medicine demands similar humility. Writers must be sensitive to what their characters want, not what we think they want. Similarly, physicians must recognize, and accept, the many possible endings a patient's story might take, and why the narrative could take that direction. Any conflict shouldn't be ignored, deemphasized or mechanically handled but probed and pulled apart.

(p. 468)

Both creative writers and health professionals must initially reside in disorganized stories. Creative writers ask questions of fictional characters, and health professionals ask questions of patients, that allow them to reveal their identity, motivations, and desires. As fictional characters and patients divulge their stories, the organizing schema of the drama and the illness become clearer and infused with meaning.

COPING SKILLS: PROBABILITY STATISTICS, EVIDENCE-BASED MEDICINE, TRUST, SHARED DECISION MAKING

The European Association for Quality in General Practice/Family Medicine (EQuiP) (2011) recommends health professional students receive education that specifically targets coping skills for working in the uncertain healthcare environment. To build coping skills, EQuiP recommends educational programming that underscores the application of population-level probability statistics to individual patients; use of evidence-based medicine when possible while allowing for the individual patient's sociocultural influences, beliefs, and values; emphasis on a trusting health professional–patient relationship; and engaging the patient in shared decision making. Shared decision making is discussed in detail in the next section.

DECISION MAKING

A decision is a choice made from among options. All of us make hundreds of decisions each day, often with little thought and minimal consequence. The stakes are raised, however, in the healthcare arena. I am not referring to decisions made in an emergency situation. Emergencies require a health professional to make rapid, unilateral decisions based on his or her understanding of the patient's condition and the prevailing evidence and standard of care. Instead, the focus of this section is on the plethora of insoluble medical scenarios that involve a range of options leading to uncertain, risky, and/or irrevocable outcomes. Some examples include scenarios in which decisions must be made about surgical interventions, use of ventilator support, or participation in clinical trials. These medical scenarios are often values sensitive and can lead to decisional conflict for patients and families, as well as health professionals. Decisional conflict is the intrapersonal psychological discomfort one experiences when there is no clear course of action, and the available choices involve ill-defined probability, dispute one's personal values, and potentially lead to immutable loss (Kattan, 2009).

WHAT CONSTITUTES A GOOD DECISION?

Before we further investigate decision making, let's establish what constitutes a "good" decision? The late professor of surgery, Richard Dow, MD (1999), from Geisel School of Medicine at Dartmouth College, described three criteria for a good decision: 1) informed by facts; 2) practical to implement; and 3) compatible with the patient's values. Dr. Dow's criteria align with sociologic models of decision making which balance rational thinking with the broader social context in which we consider risk and manage uncertainty in the process of making a decision (Bruch & Feinberg, 2017). Next, we look in detail at each of the three criteria for a good decision while noting social environments, interactions, and influences.

INFORMED BY FACTS

The first criterion of a good decision is that it must be informed by facts. Keep in mind that for many of us, facts are malleable and easily distorted by bias, emotion (especially fear), and case reports. Among patients, case reports primarily derive from the experiences of family, friends and neighbors with similar conditions. The Pew Research Center conducted a nationwide survey of 3,014 US adults living with a chronic disease (Fox & Duggan, 2013). Results found 65% of respondents report using family and friends as a central resource for health information. This is in contrast to 59% of respondents who report using the internet to find information about a specific medical condition.

Health professionals must retain responsibility for educating patients so, as much as possible, patients can make decisions informed by quality evidence. That said, health professionals' knowledge base can be prejudiced by a host of factors, some of which are described in chapter 3 Unconscious Bias, and two factors, availability bias and confirmatory bias, which are described briefly here.

AVAILABILITY BIAS AND CONFIRMATORY BIAS

Clinical decision making is subject to error originating in health professional bias. One such error, *availability heuristics* or *availability bias*, arises from our recent experiences with our patients (Croskerry, 2003; Klein, 2005). A specific consequence of availability bias is that we are inclined to diagnosis Patient D with the same disease we saw in Patients A,

B, and C, with little regard for Patient D's signs and symptoms indicating other possible diagnoses (Mamede et al., 2010). Similarly, if one of our patients develops adverse side effects from an intervention, we are less inclined to offer that intervention to another patient – independent of the evidence base for the intervention's effectiveness. Another error, *confirmatory bias*, stems from our active quest to identify physical examination findings which confirm our pre-determined diagnosis, while ignoring or dismissing findings that contradict our expectations (Kahneman, Slovic, & Tversky, 1982). In other words, we find what we want to find.

Whether we are patients or health professionals, the experiences of people we know, as well as our personal prejudices, powerfully influence the decision-making process. Health professionals have an obligation to recognize and overcome availability bias and confirmatory bias since these types of representative heuristics can corrupt our diagnostic and decision-making aptitude.

PRACTICAL TO IMPLEMENT: A PATIENT CASE

Secondly, a good decision must be practical to implement. This means it must be affordable, efficacious, geographically accessible, and integrate the patient's social support system. To get a better sense of the practical component of a good decision, let's look at a clinical case. An 80-year-old man lives alone and is adamant that he wants to remain at home. He has progressive chronic renal failure that now requires dialysis three times per week. He also has severe arthritis of the hands that effectively precludes fine motor control. He has one daughter who lives two hours away and visits every weekend. Her work and family responsibilities do not allow her to visit during the week. The daughter cleans her dad's home, does his laundry, prepares meals for the week, and tends to his finances. He socializes with a few friends in town, all of whom are dealing with age-related disabilities. The patient and daughter read online about home peritoneal dialysis and decide that it is the best course of action to support his renal failure. Unfortunately, the arthritis in his hands prohibits the patient from safely operating the dialysis machine at home by himself. The daughter's other responsibilities make it impossible for her to manage her dad's dialysis three times per week. Unless they can identify someone who the patient feels comfortable having in his home three times per week to help with dialysis and who is physically and cognitively capable of the tasks, then peritoneal dialysis at home does not meet the practical to implement criterion for a good decision.

COMPATIBLE WITH PATIENT'S VALUES

The third criterion for a good decision is compatibility with the patient's values. Columbia University professor of medicine, Rita Charon, MD, PhD (2006, p. 177), contextualizes the role of illness and the health professional in guiding patients to elucidate their values.

> Sickness opens doors. It may not always have been the case, but today, it is more likely to be sickness than, say, the loss of faith that propels a person toward self-knowledge and clarifying of life goals and values. It is when you are sick that you have to question whom in your life you trust, how much life means to you, how much

suffering you can bear. It is more likely to be the doctor than the priest or confessor who hears the answers to these questions. Illness and body state have eclipsed other life events as that which defines individuals to themselves, first of all, and then to those around them.

Illness drives a person to confront the existential questions of life and define the values that provide succor. The compassionate, aware health professional who is trained in history receiving is perfectly situated to shepherd the patient's value-definition process (see chapter 2 Patient as Storyteller: Determinants of Health). Let's look at a clinical communication tool that health professionals can use to facilitate the patient's values-definition process.

CLINICAL COMMUNICATION TOOL – ETHNICS

As discussed in chapter 1 Introduction: The Power of Story, Explanatory Model of Disease section, patient values tend to be informed by culture, family, and religion (Kleinman, 1988). There are several clinical communication tools derived from Kleinman's Explanatory Model of Disease that augment the clinical history and help health professionals explore influential, values-laden constructs with patients. One such model is ETHNIC, which stands for Explanation, Treatment, Healers, Negotiate, Intervention, Collaborate (Levin, Like, & Gottlieb, 2000). A subsequent publication added an S to the ETHNIC mnemonic to remind clinicians to include spirituality in their discussion with senior patients (Kobylarz, Heath, & Like, 2002). Table 8.1 presents sample queries and probes for each of the ETHNICS elements.

Once the patient's values are expressed, the health professional must be diligent to integrate those values into treatment decisions. Even when the patient's values conflict with the health professional's values, the self-aware health professional can still play a vital role in helping the patient reconcile his or her values with the realities of choice.

On the flip side, there is evidence that health professionals' beliefs and values influence the care provided to patients. A novel study conducted by the European Ethicus Study Group looked at physicians' religious affiliations and culture, and the end-of-life decisions they made in the intensive care unit (Sprung et al., 2007). The study population included adult patients (N = 3,086) admitted to 37 intensive care units across 17 countries in Europe who required end-of-life care decisions. For the purpose of the study, end-of-life care decisions were categorized as cardiopulmonary resuscitation (CPR), withholding life-sustaining treatment (WH), withdrawing life-sustaining treatment (WD), and active shortening of the dying process (SDP). The proxy variable for culture was the geographic region (Northern, Central, Southern) in which the intensive care unit was located in Europe. The study patients and their attending physicians identified as Catholic, Protestant, Jewish, Greek Orthodox, Muslim, No Affiliation, or Other. The authors report,

Table 8.1 ETHNICS questions and probes

Direct questions / statements	Probes
EXPLANATION	
Why do you think you have this . . . (symptom/illness/condition)?	What do friends, family, and others say about these symptoms? Do you know anyone else who has this kind of problem? Have you heard about/read/seen it on television/radio/newspaper/internet?
TREATMENT	
What have you tried for this . . . (symptom/illness/condition)?	What kind of medicines, home remedies, or other treatments have you tried for this illness? Is there anything you eat, drink, or do (or avoid) on a regular basis to stay healthy? What kind of treatments are you seeking from me?
HEALERS	
Who else have you sought help from for this . . . (symptom/illness/condition)?	Have you sought help from alternative or folk healers, friends, or other people for your problems?
NEGOTIATE	
How best do you think I can help you?	Try to find options that will be mutually acceptable to you and your patient and that incorporate your patient's beliefs rather than contradicting them.
INTERVENTION	
This is what I think needs to be done now.	Determine an intervention with your patient that may also incorporate alternative treatments, spirituality, healers, and other cultural practices.
COLLABORATE	
How can we work together on this? Who else should be involved?	Collaborate with the patient, family members, healers, and community resources.
SPIRITUALITY	
What role does faith/religion/spirituality play in helping you with this . . . (symptom/illness/condition)?	Tell me about your spiritual life. How can your spiritual beliefs help you with your illness?

Adapted from Kobylarz, Heath, & Like, 2002. Table 1. ETNHICS: A Framework for Culturally Appropriate Geriatric Care. *Journal of the American Geriatrics Society*, 50 (9), 1584.

End of life decisions varied greatly depending on the physician's religious affiliation. Life-sustaining treatment was withheld more often than withdrawn if the physician was Jewish, Greek Orthodox, or Moslem [sic]; if physicians had no religious affiliation or were Protestant the ratio of WH/WD was about 1. Catholic physicians withdrew more often than they withheld treatment. SDP occurred only if the physician was Catholic, Protestant or had no religious affiliation, $p < 0.001$. . . .

The prevalence of CPR or limitations was similar in the North and Central regions regardless of whether the religious affiliation of the physician and the patient were the same. In the South, however, there was more CPR (53%) and fewer limitations (47%) if the religious affiliation of the physician and the patient were different than the same (29% and 71%, respectively, $p < 0.001$).

(p. 1735)

Results from this study indicate the profound influence religion and culture can have on the care that health professionals provide. It is disturbing to think that religious affiliation or non-affiliation (a demographic characteristic that most patients do not know about their health professional), may alter the course of end-of-life care. To safeguard against negatively affecting our patients' care, we must understand our own values so we can lucidly appreciate and support the values of our patients, even when they differ radically from our own. As health professionals, we must continually assess our biases, remain attentive and aware of our personal values and beliefs, and aim to make decisions that are consistent with the patient's values and best interests, rather than our own. Shared decision making, which we discuss next, is a powerful and effective way to prioritize patient values in the context of scientific evidence, while maintaining our moral compass.

SHARED DECISION MAKING

According to Charles, Gafni, and Whelan (1997), shared decision making in healthcare is a process that: 1) involves the patient and health professional, and in many cultures, the extended family as well; 2) has everyone share information with each other – typically the health professional is responsible for the technical data and the patient and/or family is responsible for stating value preferences; 3) has all involved commit to building consensus for a decision; and 4) reaches agreement between the patient and health professional (and when appropriate, the family) on the treatment plan. As you can imagine, this is a formidable undertaking. Many patients must contend with insufficient knowledge, unrealistic expectations, unclear values, family and societal pressures, paucity of support and resources, and minimal skill and self-confidence in managing voluminous information to make a decision – all the ingredients for decisional conflict (Thompson-Leduc, Turcotte, Labrecque, & Legare, 2016).

What happens when one does not contend with decisional conflict? A meta-analysis of 10 clinical trials that included a total of 1,826 study participants shows that when patients do not resolve decisional conflict there are considerable consequences (Sun, 2004). Patients with decisional conflict are 23 times more likely to delay a decision, five times more likely to have regret about their decision, and three times more likely to fail a knowledge test about their diagnosis than patients who are not experiencing decisional conflict.

DECISION SUPPORT FOR HEALTHCARE

Over the past several decades, the science of decision support for healthcare has been continually refined. A recent systematic review demonstrates the clear value of decision aids in improving knowledge and expectations, lowering decisional conflict, and increasing agreement between values and choices (Stacey et al., 2017). At present, leaders in the field point to the Ottawa Decision Support Framework as the gold standard for facilitating shared decision making (Ottawa Hospital Research Institute, 2015). The Ottawa Decision Support Framework dissects the decision-making process into clear, logical steps, namely clarifying precisely what the decision is; illuminating what is needed to make the decision; exploring one's knowledge and values related to the perceived options; identifying who one's supporters are, as well as who is hindering one's decision; and finally, planning how to overcome needs or obstacles and ultimately arrive at a decision. The Ottawa Decision Support Framework is unique among health-related decision-making frameworks in that it specifically operationalizes decisional conflict for both the patient and the health professional.

Research of patient–physician dyads wrestling with high stakes clinical decisions demonstrates that implementation of the Ottawa Decision Support Framework leads to decreased decisional conflict for all involved – patients *and* physicians (Legare, O'Connor, Graham, Wells, & Trembay, 2006). Of note, the research showed that "physician-level factors explained 31% of the variance in the difference between patients' and physicians' decisional conflict score" (p. 384). Physicians who were least comfortable with uncertainty and with sharing their uncertainty with patients experienced the highest decisional conflict. The Ottawa Decision Support Framework helped physicians and patients resolve their disagreements and achieve congruence. This study underscores the importance of mutuality between health professionals and patients (see chapter 6 Recognizing Our Interdependence).

As health professionals, when we apply our clinical skills – listening to patients, responding empathically and in a culturally humble way – we can effectively explore our patients' motivations to pursue health. With attention, effort, and skill building, health professionals can acknowledge our own uncertainty, share the decision-making journey with patients, and concurrently help resolve our, and our patients', decisional conflict. All of which leads us to secure improved clinical outcomes.

CLOSING

In this chapter, we looked at the theoretical underpinnings of uncertainty as expressed by the complex adaptive systems of health and healthcare. We examined the effect uncertainty has on health professionals, patients, and their interaction. We highlighted interventions to improve health professionals' tolerance for uncertainty. We then looked at decisions and what goes into facilitating shared decision making between health professionals and patients.

I close this chapter with learning objectives and activities that encourage the reader to critique uncertainty and decision making in the clinical setting.

ACTIVITIES

LEARNING OBJECTIVES

Learners will

1 explore the complex processes involved in making a decision;
2 recognize the role of the health professional in facilitating shared decision making;
3 reflect on their personal experience of making serious decisions.

POEM AND DISCUSSION

First, read the poem, *Tubes*, by Donald Hall (2006, p. 181). Audio and text for the poem is available at www.poemhunter.com/poem/tubes/

As you read, note words or passages that appeal to you, repel you, resonate with you, startle you, or in some way catch your attention. Drawing on material presented in chapter 8, reflect on uncertainty in healthcare and the need to make decisions within the context of uncertainty.

SMALL GROUP DISCUSSION

Learners are invited to discuss their experience with the poem. Whenever possible, learners should refer to specific passages in the poem. In particular, learners should aim to comment on uncertainty and decision making. Faculty facilitators may choose to ask someone to read aloud a passage from the poem that captured their attention. Reading aloud makes the text a presence in the room and helps everyone focus. If at all possible, allow the conversation about the text to evolve organically, directed by the learners' curiosity.

NOTE: **Appendix A** has general guidelines for facilitating a health humanities seminar. **Appendix B** has instruction and discussion prompts specific to this activity for faculty facilitators to use if your learners are not able to initiate a robust discussion.

WRITING AND SHARING

The second activity is for the learner to write to a prompt that directly links the chapter content and the short story. Here is a suggested writing prompt:

> What are your "notions of balance between extremes of fortune." Feel free to write fiction.

Faculty facilitators can invite the learners to share what they have written with the group. Learners should never be required to share their writings.

REFERENCE LIST

Baruch, J. M. (2013). Creative writing as a medical instrument. *Journal of Medical Humanities, 34*, 459–469.

Bruch, E., & Feinberg, F. (2017). Decision-making processes in social contexts. *Annual Review of Sociology, 43*, 207–227.

Charles, C., Gafni, A., & Whelan, T. (1997). Shared decision-making in the medical encounter: What does it mean? (Or it takes at least two to tango). *Social Science & Medicine, 44*(5), 681–692.

Charon, R. (2006). *Narrative medicine: Honoring the stories of illness.* New York: Oxford University Press.

Cranley, L. A., Doran, D. M., Tourangeau, A. E., Kushniruk, A., & Nagle, L. (2012). Recognizing and responding to uncertainty: A grounded theory of nurses' uncertainty. *Worldviews on Evidence-Based Nursing*, Third Quarter, 149–158.

Croskerry, P. (2003). The importance of cognitive errors in diagnosis and strategies to minimize them. *Academic Medicine, 78*(8), 775–780.

Dow, R. (1999). What is a good decision? *Effective Clinical Practice, 2*(4), 187.

European Association for Quality in General Practice/Family Medicine. (2011). Dealing with uncertainty in general practice: An essential skill for the general practitioner. *Quality in Primary Care, 19*, 175–181.

Fox, S., & Duggan, M. (2013). The diagnosis difference: A portrait of the 45% of US adults living with chronic health conditions. *Pew Research Center*. Retrieved from www.pewinternet.org/2013/11/26/the-diagnosis-difference/

Golder, S., Loke, Y. K., Wright, K., & Norman, G. (2016). Reporting adverse events in published and unpublished studies of health care interventions: A systematic review. *PLoS Medicine, 13*, e1002127. doi:10.1371/journal.pmed.1002127

Hall, D. (2006). *White apples and the taste of stone.* Boston, MA: Houghton Mifflin.

Han, P. K. J., Klein, W. M. P., & Arora, N. K. (2011). Varieties of uncertainty in health care: A conceptual taxonomy. *Medical Decision Making, 31*(6), 828–838.

Heath, I. (2013). Complexity, uncertainty and mess as the links between science and the humanities in health care. In J. P. Sturmberg & C. M. Martin (Eds.), *Handbook of systems and complexity in health* (pp. 19–24). New York: Springer.

Hillen, M. A., Cutheil, C. M., Strout, T. D., Smets, E. M. A., & Han, P. K. J. (2017). Tolerance of uncertainty: Conceptual analysis, integrative model, and implications for healthcare. *Social Science & Medicine, 180,* 62–75.

Iannelo, P., Mottini, A., Tirelli, S., Riva, S., & Antonietti, A. (2017). Ambiguity and uncertainty tolerance, need for cognition, and their association with stress. A study among Italian practicing physicians. *Medical Education Online, 22*(1), 1270009. doi:1 0.1080/10872981.2016.1270009

Kahneman, D., Slovic, P., & Tversky, A. (Eds.). (1982). *Judgement under uncertainty: Heuristics and biases.* Cambridge: Cambridge University Press.

Kattan, M. W. (Ed.). (2009). *Encyclopedia of medical decision making.* Thousand Oaks, CA: Sage.

Klein, J. G. (2005). Five pitfalls in decisions about diagnosis and prescribing. *BMJ, 330*(7494), 781–783.

Kleinman, A. (1988). *The illness narratives: Suffering, healing, and the human condition.* New York: Basic Books.

Kobylarz, F. A., Heath, J. M., & Like, R. C. (2002). The ETHNIC(S) mnemonic: A clinical tool for ethnogeriatric education. *Journal of the American Geriatrics Society, 50*(9), 1582–1589.

Kuipers, P., Kendall, E., Ehrlich, C., McIntyre, M., Barber, L., Amsters, D., . . . Brownie, S. (2011). *Complexity and health care: Health practitioner workforce, services, roles, skills and training to respond to patients with complex needs.* Brisbane, AU: Clinical Education and Training Queensland. Retrieved from www.health.qld.gov.au/__data/ assets/pdf_file/0027/150768/complexcarefull1.pdf

Lauriola, M., Foschi, R., Mosca, O., & Weller, J. (2016). Attitude toward ambiguity: Empirically robust factors in self-report personality scales. *Assessment, 23*(3), 353–373.

Legare, F., O'Connor, A. M., Graham, I. D., Wells, G. A., & Trembay, S. (2006). Impact of the Ottawa Decision Support Framework on the agreement and the difference between patients' and physicians' decisional conflict. *Medical Decision Making, 26*(4), 373–390.

Levin, S. J., Like, R. C., & Gottlieb, J. E. (2000). ETHNIC: A framework for culturally competent clinical practice. In Appendix: Useful clinical interviewing mnemonics. *Patient Care, 34,* 188–189.

Lipshitz, R., & Strauss, O. (1997). Coping with uncertainty: A naturalistic decision-making analysis. *Organizational Behavior and Human Decision Processes*, *69*(92), 149–163.

Mamede, S., van Gog, T., Rikers, R. M. J. P., van Saase, J. L. C. M., van Guldener, C., & Schmidt, H. G. (2010). Effect of availability bias and reflective reasoning on diagnostic accuracy among internal medicine residents. *JAMA*, *304*(11), 1198–1203.

Mishel, M. H. (1981). The measurement of uncertainty in illness. *Nursing Research*, *30*(5), 258–263.

Mishel, M. H. (1983). Adjusting the fit: Development of uncertainty scales for specific clinical populations. *Western Journal of Nursing Research*, *5*(4), 355–370.

Mishel, M. H. (1988). Uncertainty in illness. *Image: Journal of Nursing Scholarship*, *4*, 225–232.

Mishel, M. H. (1991). Reconceptualization of the uncertainty in illness theory. *Image: Journal of Nursing Scholarship*, *22*(4), 256–262.

Mukherjee, S. (2015). *The laws of medicine: Field notes from an uncertain science.* New York: Simon & Schuster, TED.

Ofri, D. (2017). Medical humanities: The rx for uncertainty? *Academic Medicine*, *92*(12), 1657–1658.

Ottawa Hospital Research Institute, (2015). *Patient decision aids.* Author. Retrieved from https://decisionaid.ohri.ca/odsf.html

Penrod, J. (2007). Living with uncertainty: Concept advancement. *Journal of Advanced Nursing*, *57*(6), 658–667.

Portnoy, D. B., Han, P. K. J., Ferrer, R. A., Klein, W. M. P., & Clauser, S. B. (2013). Physicians' attitudes about communicating and managing scientific uncertainty differ by perceived ambiguity aversion of their patients. *Health Expectations*, *16*(4), 362–372.

Schneider, A., Lowe, B., Barie, S., Joos, S., Engeser, P., & Szecsenyi, J. (2010). How do primary care doctors deal with uncertainty in making diagnostic decisions? *Journal of Evaluation in Clinical Practice*, *16*, 431–437.

Simpkin, A., & Schwartzstein, R. M. (2016). Tolerating uncertainty – the next medical revolution? *New England Journal of Medicine*, *375*(18), 1713–1715.

Sprung, C. L., Maia, P., Bulow, H., Ricou, B., Armaganidis, A., Baras, M., . . . Thijs, L. G. (2007). The importance of religious affiliation and culture on end-of-life decisions in European intensive care units. *Intensive Care Medicine, 33,* 1732–1739.

Stacey, D., Légaré, F., Lewis, K., Barry, M. J., Bennett, C. L., Eden, K. B., . . . Trevena, L. (2017). Decision aids for people facing health treatment or screening decisions. *Cochrane Database Systematic Review, 4,* CD001431. doi:10.1002/14651858. CD001431.pub5

Starr, P. (2013). Law and the fog of healthcare: Complexity and uncertainty in the struggle over health policy. *Saint Louis University Journal of Health Law & Policy, 6*(2), 213–228.

Sturmberg, J. P., & Martin, C. M. (2013). Complexity in health: An introduction. In J. P. Sturmberg & C. M. Martin (Eds.), *Handbook of systems and complexity in health* (pp. 1–17). New York: Springer.

Sun, Q. (2004). *Predicting downstream effects of high decisional conflict: Meta-analyses of the decisional conflict scale.* University of Ottawa. Retrieved from https://ruor.uottawa.ca/bitstream/10393/27050/1/MR11422.PDF

Thompson-Leduc, P., Turcotte, S., Labrecque, M., & Legare, F. (2016). Prevalence of clinically significant decisional conflict: An analysis of five studies on decision-making in primary care. *BMJ Open, 6,* e011490. doi:10.1136/bmjopen-2016-011490

Truong, Q. A., Murphy, S. A., McCabe, C. H., Armani, A., & Cannon, C. P. (2011). Benefit of intensive statin therapy in women: Results from PROVE IT-TIMI 22. *Circulation: Cardiovascular Quality and Outcomes, 4,* 3328–3336.

Unnikrishnana, M. K. (2017). Eminence or evidence? The volatility, uncertainty, complexity, and ambiguity in healthcare. *Journal of Pharmacology and Pharmacotherapeutics, 8*(1), 1–2. doi:10.4103/jpp.JPP1217

Vaismoradi, M., Salsali, M., & Ahmadi, F. (2011). Nurses' experiences of uncertainty in clinical practice: A descriptive study. *Journal of Advanced Nursing, 67*(5), 991–999.

9 PROFESSIONAL IDENTITY: PERSPECTIVES, ROLES, VALUES, AND ATTRIBUTES

> INTEGRATION NOTE
> ....
>
> This chapter integrates with clinical science education related to human development, as well as health professional well-being. The learner activities at the end of the chapter align with curriculum content related to sickle cell disease.

INTRODUCTION

Our identity is our way of knowing who we are. If you look back on your life, you may notice that your identity has shifted over time. Perhaps as a child you enjoyed your identity as class clown, book worm, or athlete. Maybe your identity was defined by your family or, if you were not a member of the dominant culture within your community, your identity was defined by your racial, ethnic, and/or religious group. As you became a young adult perhaps your identity was defined more by your accomplishments and affiliations. You became the one who works in the lab, volunteers at the hospital, attends university, is a member of the socialist party, or joined the military. You might also be identified by your relationships – you are someone's child, partner, spouse, parent, friend. At some point as an adult, you begin to define the parameters by which you identify yourself and definitively lay claim to your personal identity. Educator and activist, Parker Palmer, PhD writes,

> By identity I mean an evolving nexus where all the forces that constitute my life converge in the. . . . Self: my genetic makeup . . . the culture in which I was raised, people who have sustained me and people who have done me harm, the good and ill I have done to others, and to myself, the experience of love and suffering. . . . In the midst of that complex field, identity is a moving intersection of the inner and outer forces that make me who I am.
>
> (Palmer & Scribner, 2007, p. 108)

Why is identity of interest to health professionals? Most, if not all, of the health professional organizations express interest in promotion and cultivation of professional identity as part of their educational programming (Abreu, 2006; Cooke, Irby, O'Brien, & Shulman, 2010; Sahrmann, 2014; Ten Hoeve, Jansen, & Roodbol, 2014; Webb, 2017). Professional identity formation of healthcare workers is vital if we are to successfully fulfill our responsibilities. It is incumbent on health professionals to use our privilege of higher education and the benefit of our patients' trust and respect, to resist the role of biomedical technician and instead view ourselves as humanitarians and agents of social change. Our professional identity encompasses our perspectives, roles, values, and attributes. A critical prerequisite to adopting a professional identity is comprehensive understanding of one's personal identity – thus allowing the personal and professional to integrate.

In this chapter, I look at identity from several perspectives – Western philosophy, Buddhist philosophy, psychology, and sociocultural influences. I use multiple perspectives on identity to discern the influences on our personal identity, and the relationship between our personal and professional identity. I explore components of professional identity, and the experiences of health professionals who are racial, ethnic, and/or sexual minorities. Finally, I discuss the challenges to professional identity imposed by inter-professional education and practice. I close the chapter with exercises that provide opportunity for experiential learning related to identity, perspective, and role.

PERSPECTIVES ON PERSONAL IDENTITY

Identity is a slippery concept that has vexed philosophers, psychologists, and social scientists for centuries. As foundation for our conversation on professional identity, I provide a cursory review of some of the scholarly thinking on identity that specifically relates to healthcare workers.

WESTERN PHILOSOPHY

Within metaphysical philosophy, ongoing discussion in the literature related to identity focuses on three questions:

The identification question: What properties must a being have to count as a person?

The reidentification question: What makes a person the same person over time?

The characterization question: What makes a person the person that she is?

(Kind, 2015, p. 3)

These questions are not intellectual exercises, but rather have practical applications in healthcare and biomedical ethics. Every day, health professionals, patients with life-altering illness, and their family members wrestle with the idea of personhood in order to make difficult decisions such as whether to engage life-prolonging treatment (Quante, 2017). Health professionals explore with the patient (and more often than not, with the patient's family) the effect disease renders on his or her personal identity. We delve into questions such as: Is the person you were before the disease or injury still present? Now that disease or injury has affected your ability to think, move, relate to another being . . . what makes you the person that you are?

Let's look at each of the three metaphysical philosophy identity questions in detail.

THE IDENTIFICATION QUESTION

The identification question examines the specific properties an entity must possess to be a person. In the literature you will find arguments in support of properties such as mental capacity, self-consciousness, ability to experience emotions, pleasure, and pain, consciousness of time, ability to communicate in some form, and capacity to exercise freedom of will. You will also find arguments that systematically debunk these same properties by demonstrating how large swaths of humanity, namely infants, young children, and individuals with severe cognitive impairment, cannot demonstrate the properties of a person and yet still have undeniable personal identity (Kind, 2015; Quante, 2017). Philosophers continue to work on the identification question: some raise the idea of potential persons for infants and young children who cannot yet demonstrate the properties but have the potential to do so over time. Others posit that the essential essence of personhood still awaits classification (Madell, 2015). Still others, like Oxford University philosopher, Derek Parfit (1984), take a reductionist approach to personal identity arguing that people exist as a composite of components (i.e., body, cognition, and memory) and interconnections with other people. Parfit goes so far as to say that personal identity does not matter since individuals are essentially social constructs. According to Parfit, interpersonal connectedness takes primacy over personal identity. As described in chapter 6 Recognizing Our Interdependence and the Buddhist Philosophy section below, Parfit's emphasis on interconnectedness has roots in Buddhism.

THE RE-IDENTIFICATION QUESTION

The re-identification question, what makes a person the same person over time, is a persistent puzzle for philosophers. The aim is to establish if my personal identity as a 55-year-old professor is the same as when I was a 45-year-old research scientist, a 30-year-old physician assistant, and a 5-year-old child? What are the metaphysical criteria that demonstrate the continued existence of my personhood over time? In his 1689 germinal text, *An Essay Concerning Human Understanding*, philosopher John Locke (1996, p. 138) wrote,

> This being premised to find wherein *personal identity* consists, we must consider what *person* stands for; which, I think, is a thinking intelligent being, that has reason and reflection, and can consider itself as itself, the same thinking thing in different times and places; which it does only by that consciousness, which is inseparable from thinking, and as it seems to me essential to it: it being impossible for anyone to perceive, without perceiving, that he does perceive. When we see, hear, smell, taste, feel, meditate, or will anything, we know that we do so. Thus it is always as to our present sensations and perceptions: and by this everyone is to himself, that which he calls *self*: it not being considered in this case, whether the same *self* be continued in the same, or divers [sic] substances. For since consciousness always accompanies thinking, and 'tis that, that makes everyone to be, what he calls *self*; and thereby distinguishes himself from all other thinking things, in this alone consists *personal*

identity, i.e. the sameness of a rational being: and as far as this consciousness can be extended backwards to any past action or thought, so far reaches the identity of that *person*; it is the same *self* now it was then; and 'tis by the same *self* with this present one that now reflects on it, that that action was done. [italics in original text]

With this passage, Locke positions personal identity as a function of memory ("consciousness extended backward to any past action or thought") and the embodied experience, thereby distinguishing identity from the spiritual realm of soul. Referred to as Locke's Memory Theory of Personal Identity, the premise asserts if a person can remember an experience then that person had the experience – and the converse – if a person cannot remember an experience then that person did not have that experience. Let's think about Locke's Theory for a moment. It implies that you are not the same person as you were as a toddler, simply because you have no conscious memory of that time in your life. This leads us to the question – do people with dementia have no connection to the self who has experiences they cannot remember because of their disease? What about people who experience trauma resulting in amnesia to the traumatic event – does the fact that they do not remember the trauma mean that it happened to someone else? How does Locke's Theory account for sleep, anesthesia, or inebriated states that someone cannot remember the next day?

Modern philosophers have iteratively critiqued and modified Locke's Memory Theory to account for discontinuous memory while still maintaining the intent of the theory. The modified theory asserts that continuity of memory does not mean the memories must be present in the mind, but rather that they have the potential to occur (Kind, 2015). In practical language this means that although my 55-year-old self may not remember the experiences of my 2-year-old self, my memories (and in turn, my personhood) are considered continuous if my 55-year-old self remembers the experiences of my 20-year-old self, and my 20-year-old self remembers the experiences of my 10-year-old self, who remembers my 5-year-old self experiences, who remembers my 2-year-old self experiences. The assertion of potential occurrence is helpful, however, it still does not explicate the connection to periods of time when memory of experiences are obliterated. There are philosophers who reject the memory theory in favor of psychological or bodily approaches to personal identity, or what is called Further Fact View, or a hybrid view that encompasses components of multiple approaches (Brison, 2002). At present there is no consensus position on re-identification. Needless to say, philosophers continue to pursue the answer to the question, what makes a person the same person over time?

THE CHARACTERIZATION QUESTION

The third personal identity question seeks to characterize what makes us who we are. In the text, *Staying Alive: Personal Identity, Practical Concerns, and the Unity of a Life*, University of Illinois, Chicago philosophy professor Marya Schechtman, PhD (2014) presents the Person Life View of personal identity. Person Life View defines key factors that are essential for a person to define the characteristic life she or he leads. Professor Schechtman (p. 137) writes,

A paradigmatic person life is a characteristic developmental trajectory that can be understood on three interconnected levels: the level of capabilities and attributes, the level of activities and interactions, and the level of social infrastructure.

Let's look at the three levels Professor Schechtman refers to – capabilities and attributes, activities and interactions, and social infrastructure – in more detail. The capabilities and attributes level refers to the physical and psychological capacities that the individual has, including bodily strength and stamina, intellectual prowess, and emotional competency. The activities and interactions level encompasses the application of an individual's capabilities and attributes to survive and potentially thrive in daily life. The social infrastructure level refers to the environment, culture, and institutions that support or denigrate the activities and interactions of an individual within a community. Professor Schechtman compares Person Life View to the biological case for human life which includes functioning organ systems, metabolic activities, and a plethora of complex interactions, each of which are necessary but none of which are individually sufficient to maintain the health of the individual. Similarly, biological, psychological, and social features, which manifest as capabilities, attributes, activities, inter-relations, and social infrastructure, intertwine to create personal identity.

The philosophical argument for the crucial interdependence among biological, psychological, and social features necessary for personal identity are a profound reminder of the need for comprehensive whole person healthcare. As described in chapter 2 Patient as Storyteller, Determinants of Health section, Healthy People 2020 (2018) identifies four categories that determine an individual's health: biology and genetics, individual behavior, social and physical environment, and health services. The considerable overlap between the Person Life View features and the Healthy People 2020 health determinants indicates personal identity is an essential element of health.

BUDDHIST PHILOSOPHY

Foundational to Buddhism is the concept of non-self, which by its very definition defies the idea of personal identity. Non-self does not mean that we do not exist – rather, non-self refers to the notion that all life is interconnected and arises from unified energy. The individual only exists in relationship to everyone and everything else (see chapter 6 Recognizing Our Interdependence), all of which is continually changing. Of note, Buddhist philosophy describes humans as a consortium of the physical body, feelings, perceptions, responses, and consciousness – which is remarkably similar to the list of personal identity properties that Western philosophers ascribe (see earlier). However, from a Buddhist perspective the consortium is constantly changing and insubstantial, and therefore, neither attainable nor identifiable (Emmanuel, 2013). When we attempt to identify with a particular pattern of properties within our body or mind, we grasp at an impermanent illusion. Each point of attachment where we might claim personal identity, such as our relationships, our occupation, or our home, is invariably transient and will die or change, in time. Even our thoughts and feelings, which seem so intimate and personal, change according to conditions. Think about your own experiences – you are not consumed by a single thought or emotion for a sustained period of time. Anger, joy, loneliness, curiosity, fear, and more, arise and dissipate depending on conditions (Kornfield, 1993).

While Western philosophers recognize the transience of personal identity (see The Re-identification Question section), they remain committed to finding a lasting identity over time. Buddhist philosophers, on the other hand, recognize the transience of all things, including personal identity, and concurrently realize the generativity of interconnectedness and emptiness that give rise to all. The Buddhist concept of non-self liberates us from the confines of socially and culturally constructed ideas of identity and what it means to lead a successful life (Kopf, 2015).

The Tao Te Ching is a 6th-century text that is foundational to Taoism and greatly influenced Buddhist philosophy. A modern translation of the Tao Te Ching offers a lyrical synopsis of freedom from striving for personal identity.

> Brim-fill the bowl, it'll spill over. Keep sharpening the blade, you'll soon blunt it.
>
> Nobody can protect a house full of gold and jade. Wealth, status, pride are their own ruin.
>
> To do good, work well, and lie low is the way of the blessing.
>
> (Le Guin, 1998, p. 12)

PSYCHOLOGY OF IDENTITY

Similar to the Western philosophy scholars, psychology researchers have struggled to definitively capture personal identity. As we look at the established psychological theories of personal identity, you will notice considerable overlap with Western philosophical arguments and Buddhist philosophy. We start our inquiry with Erik Erikson's Psychosocial Theory of Development. Erikson (1968) purports that across the life span we are presented with conflicts or crises that lead us to "a crucial period of increased vulnerability and heightened potential." Erikson goes on to say that individuals re-emerge "from each crisis with an increased sense of inner unity, with an increase of good judgment, and an increase in the capacity 'to do well' according to his own standards and to the standards of those who are significant to him" (p 91). In other words, our conflicts, crises, and challenges are opportunities for self-revelation of our true identity. By including the phrase "according to his own standards and the standards of those who are significant to him," Erikson firmly situates identity formation within a sociocultural context. This is an important conceptualization that has endured for decades and spawned sociocultural identity and narrative identity theories (see Sociocultural Influences section that follows).

Erikson was one of the first theorists to describe personal identity in terms of a coherent self that persists through time, environmental change, and altered roles (Sokol, 2009). He places three domains at the cornerstone of an individual's personal identity: fidelity,

BOX 9.1

A few years ago, I attended a training on end-of-life care at Upaya Institute and Zen Center in Sante Fe, New Mexico led by Frank Ostaseski, founder of the Zen Hospice Program and Metta Institute, and Roshi Joan Halifax, anthropologist and founder and Abbot of the Upaya Institute and Zen Center. The training included a guided meditation that invited us to continually evaluate who we are as we systematically lose our occupation, home, friends, family, bodily functions, and body. For me, this was a profound experiential teaching on personal identity, professional identity, and non-self. If you would like to experience a similar guided meditation, I refer you to the book, *Facing Death and Finding Hope: A Guide to the Emotional and Spiritual Care of the Dying*, by Christine Longaker (1997).

The American Association of Colleges of Nursing (n.d.), End-of-Life Nursing Education Consortium, also offers powerful experiential teachings on identity. In one exercise, entitled *Eight Gifts*, participants are asked to identify their life's gifts, namely their closest friend, closest relative, dearest place, most important role, favorite activity, favorite food, current address, and their profession. As participants imagine themselves experiencing progressive life-threatening illness, they feel what it is like to have to give up one gift after another. By simulating cumulative loss, participants hope to gain appreciation for the circumstances of their patients at end of life. In my opinion, the exercise is also an opportunity to reflect upon our personal identity and values, and to consider what aspects of our personhood endure.

ideology, and work (Erikson, 1964). Fidelity refers to the commitment an individual makes to a group or ideas, typically based on a value system. Ideology refers to the belief system an individual adopts. Work refers to the occupation an individual chooses as a way of expressing personal identity and contributing to society. Erikson's foundational work on personal identity provides a readily accessible link between personal identity and professional identity, which we will discuss in more detail later in this chapter (see the Professional Identity section that follows).

Professor of Psychology at California State University, Fresno, Robert Levine, PhD (2016), uses his text, *Stranger in the Mirror: The Scientific Search for Self*, to present four themes related to personal identity. Professor Levine draws from a vast literature to posit: 1) the individual self is difficult to distinguish from one's environment and social context; 2) a person's body, mind, and actions interweave and at times are in conflict with each other; 3) each person is in a constant state of flux; and 4) evidence indicates there is no true personal identity, but rather we are pure potential always in a state of becoming. The linkages between Professor Levine's four themes and Buddhist philosophy are apparent, in particular when discussing non-individuation and the continual state of change for our bodies and minds.

Using humor and self-deprecation, Professor Levine reviews common English phrases that imply we are multiple entities within a single individual. For example, phrases like "I'm not myself today," "I scare myself," and "I hate myself" indicate there are two beings: "I" the noun and "myself" the object. "It's as if a stranger shares one's cranium, a cohabitant. The other one is me, of course, – who else could he be? – but at the same time he feels outside my control. He goes about his business with very much a mind of his own" (p. 157).

In the text, *Identity Flexibility in Adulthood: Perspectives in Adult Development*, Towson University psychology professor, Jan Sinnott, PhD (2017), presents a complex argument for knowing the evolving self at the intersection of cognition, emotion, social factors, and spiritual beliefs. Professor Sinnott refers to this intersection as the transforming self, and argues for a personal identity that is simultaneously unified and continually evolving. "This concept of identity involves no permanent fixed quality; yet it is *felt* to be stable in an ongoing way" (p. 21). Synthesizing ideas from a broad array of scientific fields, Professor Sinnott offers a comprehensive model for personal identity in adulthood that is constructed from multi-directional influences among a person's cognition, sense of connection, perception of time and finitude, memory of younger self, and personal need to create meaning in the present that will endure into the future. There is strong alignment with Buddhist thought, especially around the ideas of impermanence and connection. While Professor Sinnott avows impermanence, she also accepts standard psychological theory that human behavior typically follows a predictable pattern predicated on past behavior.

SOCIOCULTURAL INFLUENCES

We have already heard from Western philosophers, Buddhist philosophers, and psychology researchers who endorse the sociocultural influences on personal identity. To get a deeper sense of sociocultural impact, it may be helpful to think about your own life and the ways your identity is influenced by your environment, culture, and social network. Particularly in the United States, we like to think of ourselves as independent agents; however, when we reflect on our circumstances, we often see the influences of others. In many ways, we find that we are a *product of our environment*. For example, some of us pattern our adult lives after our parents, while others deliberately design lives that our antithetical to our parents. Either way, our parents and other ancestors tend to have weighty influence on our personal identity.

Dialogical theorists state that influence is imposed by everyone with whom we are in dialogue – that is, each person that we engage affects our self-perception and self-awareness and in turn is affected by us.

> The dialogical self is "social", not in the sense that a self-contained individual enters into social interactions with other outside people, but in the sense that other people occupy positions in a multivoiced self. The self is not only "here" but also "there", and, owing to the power of imagination, the person can act as if he or she were the other and the other were him- or herself.
>
> (Hermans, 2001, p. 250)

Perhaps you have had the experience of hearing a parent's or teacher's voice in your head, guiding you through a challenging circumstance – or providing an oppositional opinion that motivates you to repudiate his or her stance and actively organize a new viewpoint.

There exists a dynamic interplay between sociocultural processes, such as societal norms and values, and an individual person's behavior. Our drive for self-preservation and innate fear of being ostracized leads us to internalize many sociocultural processes and express them as our personal identity and personal behavior (Penuel & Wertsch, 1995). Personal identity does not arise de nova, nor is it a mechanistic recapitulation of sociocultural processes. From a sociocultural perspective, personal identity is in a constant state of redefinition as new external information is integrated with historical and biological matter.

Michigan State University philosophy professor and bioethicist, Hilde Lindemann, PhD, asserts that sociocultural containment of personhood is a moral practice. In the text, *Holding and Letting Go: The Social Practice of Personal Identities,* Professor Lindemann (2014) describes how our identity is made and maintained by the activities of other people. Focusing on individuals with severe cognitive impairment, Professor Lindemann outlines the moral practice of family caregivers who hold the impaired individual in personhood by using stories and other intimate exchanges. You may recall from Locke's Memory Theory of Personal Identity (described in the Western Philosophy section), individuals with severe cognitive impairment are unable to meet criteria for personhood, primarily because they are unable to form and connect to memories of their experiences. Drawing from encounters within her own family, Professor Lindemann provides a thoughtful and comprehensive argument for personhood being created and held by one's social network through stories. This leads us to discussion of Narrative Identity Theory.

NARRATIVE IDENTITY THEORY

Narrative Identity Theory is a subset of sociocultural identity that prioritizes the impact of stories – our own and others' – on personal identity. In the text, *The Co-Authored Self: Family Stories and the Construction of Personal Identity,* professor of psychology at Western Washington University, Kate McLean (2016, p. 20) writes,

> A personal identity is constructed not only in the weaving together of a person's own experiences into coherent narratives, but also in the weaving together of multiple layers of narratives that surround the person. As members of families, individuals have available to them a multitude of stories told by and about family members that are in play as individuals construct a storied understanding of the self.

Stories are the means by which we grow to understand our environment, culture, values, and beliefs. In addition, stories help us to make sense of our own thoughts and behaviors, and give meaning to our lives. Professor McLean (p. 5) writes,

> We are not simply autonomous agents who pick and choose the stories we select into ourselves, constructing an identity only to meet our own needs. We are also subject to the stories of others. To the stories others tell about us. To the stories others tell about themselves. Even in some cases, strange as it may sound, to the stories others *don't* tell. An identity is not the work of a sole-author, but a collaboration: the co-authored self. [italics in original text]

In part, stories allow us to manage the three formidable challenges of identification, re-identification, and characterization (see Western Philosophy section). The fragmented self and personal discontinuity that erupts when we examine our behaviors and characteristics over time and in different environments is assuaged by stories. Stories allow us to see the multiplicity of our possible selves (e.g., child, adult, parent, lover, worker, advocate, adventurer, artist, spiritual being), while simultaneously revealing qualities that endure across all these roles. Stories, and the narrative work which proliferates from them, provide a propitious forum for asking the question at the core of personal identity – who am I?

PROFESSIONAL IDENTITY

I think many health professionals would agree that our educational experiences can, at times, be a crucible. We arrive with an identity informed by our familial and sociocultural influences; however, once in our training, we encounter a new family and culture unique to healthcare that – in the presence of challenge, crisis, and vulnerability – burnishes a new identity. In his book, *A Hidden Wholeness: The Journey Toward an Undivided Life*, Parker Palmer (2004, p. 5) cautions us about dividing our personal and professional identities. "I pay a high price when I live a divided life – feeling fraudulent, anxious about being found out, and depressed by the fact that I am denying my selfhood." Palmer encourages us to find wholeness in our workplace, rejoining our personal and professional identity – what he refers to as "soul and role" (p. 21). He recommends finding a community of practice that welcomes wholeness within a "circle of trust" (p. 73). *A Hidden Wholeness* gives a detailed description of the robust programming Palmer offers health professionals and others who need to integrate personal and professional identities within a challenging work culture. He sets a high standard that appears to yield a high reward. Here is a list of the key features of the programming:

- Commit to act in concert with our conscience and values.
- Find and cultivate a culture and community of trust and support.
- Take note of our own thoughts and intentions.
- Use art, literature, music, and nature to gently expand our vision.
- Name our own truth and speak our truth clearly.
- Listen deeply.
- Commit to the Third Way: Nonviolence in everyday life.

PROFESSIONAL IDENTITY FORMATION

As a health professional student progresses to independent healthcare worker, professional identity formation is achieved primarily through socialization within the community of practice (Cruess, Cruess, Boudreau, Snell, & Steinert, 2015). During the socialization process, the healthcare system is the dominant cultural influence on the individual's professional identity, and health professionals and patients are the social network. Expectations, norms, and standards are set by the healthcare system and are undeniably different than those experienced in the larger community. For example, it is inappropriate, and in many cases illegal, to place our hands on the body of a relative stranger – and yet, within the context of healthcare, it is not only appropriate, it is required. We place our hands on another's body as professionals with the intention to help, not as laypeople seeking pleasure, power, or harm. Socialization largely happens informally during clinical training as students are exposed to health professional role models and experience feedback from patients. Ideally, conscious reflection provides the student with the opportunity to discern optimal attitudes and behaviors from role models whom they wish to emulate, as well as attitudes and behaviors that they choose to actively refrain from adopting.

We must be careful that socialization is not simply the polite word for hidden curriculum. The hidden curriculum in health professional education refers to the content and messaging that is taught without intention or awareness, and exists in contrast to the formal curriculum (Hafferty & O'Donnell, 2015). When health professional faculty display exclusionary behaviors, such as disrespect and disregard for certain patient populations, then the socialization process for students encompasses exclusionary behaviors – regardless of the faculty's intent. Faculty who fail to demonstrate empathy, or are driven by expediency and profit rather than their patients' well-being, socialize students to the same. The presence of such faculty drives a hidden curriculum that says someone can exhibit discrimination, selfishness, and paucity of emotional awareness, and still succeed in healthcare and academia. Every time we ignore unprofessional behavior among our colleagues, or make excuses for their actions, we are complicit. We add to the hidden curriculum that subverts professional identity for *unprofessional* identity and batters the heart of healthcare. As health professionals, it is imperative that we champion formal professional identity formation curriculum for our students so we can help them discern attitudes, beliefs, and behaviors that optimize their personal growth and ability to care for patients.

VALUES, COMMITMENTS, AND ASPIRATIONS

Rachel Naomi Remen, MD, founder and director of the Remen Institute for the Study of Health and Wellness, and her colleagues studied over 600 medical students who attended The Healer's Art program at 31 English-speaking medical schools (Rabow, Evans, & Remen, 2013). The purpose of the study was to identify students' beliefs about aspects of themselves that they feared would be lost during their medical training and professional identity formation as physicians. The students "were asked to reflect, identify, and draw a part of themselves that they were wary about revealing, not comfortable showing, or felt may be diminished in medical school and label this part with a word" (p. 13). Qualitative analysis revealed five thematic areas in which the students' words of concern were clustered: spirituality (sample words – hope, faith, reflection), emotional engagement (sample words – empathy, connectedness), identity/self-expression (sample words – me, wholeness), freedom/spontaneity (sample words – spontaneity, free spirit), and relationships (sample words – family, friendships). Particularly noteworthy to our discussion of professional identity is the fact that *creativity* was the most common word the students used to identify what they feared losing during their medical training. Exercises like the one used in this study help students recognize the personal qualities that they value, and commit to integrate those qualities into their professional identity.

Muriel Bebeau, PhD and Kathy Faber-Langendoen, MD (2014), in the text *Remediation in Medical Education: A Mid-course Correction*, describe three enduring components of both personal and professional identity formation: our values, commitments, and aspirations. The values component refers to beliefs or ideals that we hold precious and are desirable. Commitments are what we choose to dedicate ourselves to, the responsibilities or actions that we are devoted to achieving and maintaining. Aspirations are our dreams and hopes. Our values, commitments, and aspirations can endure through time and across circumstances, and thus supersede the impermanence of affiliative identity. When we garner a sense of our values, commitments, and aspirations – and find convergence of our personal and professional values, commitments, and aspirations – then we are well on our way to solidifying an authentic identity that honors our coherent, undivided self.

MINORITY PERSPECTIVE

Those of us who are minorities, whether by race, ethnicity, national origin, gender, gender expression, sexual orientation, religion, and/or, mobility, must learn to

BOX 9.2

Several years ago I attended the course, *Healing Healthcare Disparities through Education: An Interdisciplinary Faculty Development Program* at Harvard Medical School. Hasan Bazari, MD, internist and former internal medicine residency director at Massachusetts General Hospital, was one of the presenters. Dr. Bazari invited us to write two lists: our personal values, commitments, and aspirations, and our professional values, commitments, and aspirations. We compared the lists, looking for alignment and differences, and ways to integrate the personal and professional. We then shared our insights. The health professionals in attendance shared powerful and riveting statements that affirmed their integrity, decency, compassion, and creativity. This was a moving and valuable learning activity for me as I experienced the importance of periodically rediscovering and reclaiming our humanity and personhood, and reconnecting with others who are on the service path.

negotiate the sociocultural influences of our personal identity *plus* the influences of the dominant culture (Ting-Toomey, 2015). In order to successfully communicate and attain positive identity affirmation from members of the dominant culture, we must traverse the dialectical spectrum such that the members of the dominant culture maintain their identity security. This usually means minorities need to use language that is peppered with the norms and standards of the dominant culture. Sadly, for minority healthcare providers, this may not be enough to satisfy the dominant culture.

A nascent literature exists of personal accounts by minority health professionals who are not recognized by peers and patients, despite their education and competence. In some situations, individuals have been denied the opportunity to practice their profession. Of note, this small body of literature is composed, almost exclusively, of physician authors. Possibly other health professionals, with less perceived social and professional capital than physicians, feel too vulnerable to publish their personal experiences of discrimination and exclusion. Here are brief excerpts from publications that portray the experiences of minority health professionals.

In her *Annals of Family Medicine* essay, J. Nwando Olayiwola, MD, MPH (2016) describes the microaggressions that are part of her daily life, including not being acknowledged by the security guard at the facility where she works unless she is wearing her white coat and identification badge. Dr. Olayiwola goes on to depict her experience with a hostile patient who spews an aggressive rant about her race and gender, and refuses to allow her to touch him.

> Racism had just completely and tectonically shifted the power away from me. Racism stripped me of my white coat, my stethoscope, my doctor's badge, my degrees and credentials, my titles, my skills, and my determination to serve.
>
> (p. 268)

She shares her frustration with the inequitable standards that are set for women of color in healthcare.

> Black women (and other professional minority women) have to justify professional qualifications that should speak for themselves. We have to be "twice as" . . . good, smart, talented, aggressive, outspoken, witty, etc than everyone else in our professional or work environments; proving that we are not "imposters," biting our tongues and tempering our words because we don't want to appear "angry"; being passed up or looked over, underpaid, undervalued, and underappreciated.
>
> (p. 268)

Roberto E. Montenegro, MD, PhD (2016) writes in his *JAMA* essay about being mistaken for a valet on the very night he was celebrating completion of his dissertation.

I was at the pinnacle of my celebration, and with one swift action, I was dismissed. I was made invisible. I was negated. I had worked so hard for what I was celebrating; my body, however, fully defined me in that moment – I was lumped into a category based on my appearance, my ethnicity.

(p. 2071)

Dr. Montenegro recalls the persistent, derogatory comments he endured during his medical education.

As a medical student, I often felt marginalized from my medical community. I have been told that my name is "not American," fallen prey to being confused for support staff such as a janitor (even while wearing my white coat), and been asked questions like "Where are you really from?" or "How old were you when you moved to the United States?" or "When you're done with your training, are you going back to your country?" The greatest barb, however, was being summoned as "interpreter" by an attending physician during my surgery rounds.

"Interpreter!" he would bark out. I instantly appeared before the group and would begin to interpret.

Like most other recipients of microaggressions, I was stuck trying to decide if and how I would respond to these comments, especially in such a disproportionate power dynamic. Is he trying to help me by showcasing my language skills? Is he just trying to be funny? Am I overreacting? Will I be perceived as "the angry minority" if I speak up? At these instances, I felt helpless and powerless – there were no open conversations about racism, and I was left alone to deal with these difficult situations.

(p. 2071)

My personal experiences and those of my colleagues indicate that the exclusionary and discriminatory practices described in these essays are neither unique nor rare. At a reception, thirty minutes before I would take the stage to receive an award, two attendees handed me their empty wine glasses and sashayed away without a word. Though the encounter lasted a matter of seconds, its sting persisted – a reminder that no matter my achievements, my appearance means there are people who only see me as a subordinate present to satisfy their needs, rather than their professional peer. At a recent discussion among minority physicians about personal experiences with discrimination, a surgeon shared that she was often presumed to be from dietary services and had been ordered by patients and staff to remove dirty dinner trays. A cardiologist talked about repeatedly being mistaken for janitorial staff. A pediatrician told of parents who asked him if he was homosexual, and when he answered affirmatively, did not allow him to treat their children.

For minority health professionals, the intended and unintended insults to our personhood and professional identity are plentiful, though rarely talked about or highlighted publicly. As health professionals, it is incumbent on all of us to shift the healthcare culture toward one of inclusion and recognition of intellect, skill, dedication, and compassion.

INTER-PROFESSIONAL EDUCATION: CHALLENGES TO PROFESSIONAL IDENTITY

Inter-professional education (IPE) is purported to be the ideal format for teaching future healthcare workers to function well on interdisciplinary clinical teams and improve patient outcomes (Barr et al., 2017). According to the Centre for the Advancement of Interprofessional Education, "IPE enables two or more professions to learn with, from and about each other to improve collaborative practice and quality of care" (p. 4). Although evidential support for the benefits of inter-professional healthcare are limited (Hammick, Freeth, Koppel, Reeves, & Barr, 2007), inter-professional education remains an expected standard to be achieved by medicine, nursing, and health science educators.

Recently, researchers asked: What is the effect of inter-professional education and practice on the identity held by members of distinct health professions? Is professional identity diluted by inter-professional education and practice? (McNeil, Mitchell, & Parker, 2013) Does having a professional identity for one's distinct profession interfere with one's ability to perform as part of an interdisciplinary team? (Khalili, Orchard, Spence Laschinger, & Farah, 2013) To date, there are no definitive answers to these questions; however, it seems the more often students from different health professions are able to interact with each other during their training, the better they are able to communicate across disciplines. Better communication leads to improved patient safety, so it makes sense to persevere to find best practices for inter-professional healthcare education. When healthcare workers from different professions see the commonalities among our values, commitments, and aspirations, we may expand what Parker Palmer refers to as our "circle of trust" (see Professional Identity section) and be more open to an integrated life.

CLOSING

In this chapter, we looked at identity from the perspective of Western philosophy, Buddhist philosophy, psychology, and sociocultural influences. We examined the persuasions on our personal identity, the relationship between our personal and professional identity, and the enduring qualities that supersede affiliation. We highlighted the additional challenges that minority health professionals face, and looked at the potential burdens and benefits of inter-professional education to our professional identity formation.

I close this chapter with learning objectives and activities that challenge the reader to explore personal and professional identity in the clinical setting, and consider the difference between patients' and health professionals' perspective on roles.

ACTIVITIES

LEARNING OBJECTIVES

Learners will

1 explore the concept of identity;
2 recognize the contribution of sociocultural constructs to identity formation;
3 reflect on their personal values, commitments, and aspirations;
4 recognize the influence of perspective and role on attitudes, beliefs, and values of patients and health professionals;
5 compare and contrast patients' perspectives of healthcare and health professionals' perspectives of healthcare.

SPOKEN WORD VIDEO AND DISCUSSION

First, watch the 3+ minute spoken word video, *Sickle Cell* by Jasmine Bailey (Simmons, 2009). The video can be found at www.youtube.com/watch?v=1OKkz FlWvbA

As you watch, note words or passages that appeal to you, repel you, resonate with you, startle you, or in some way catch your attention. Drawing on material presented in chapter 9, reflect on Jasmine's personal identity and the professional identity of the health professionals that Jasmine refers to.

SMALL GROUP DISCUSSION

Learners are invited to discuss their experience with the spoken word video. Whenever possible, learners should refer to specific passages in the video. In particular, learners should aim to comment on personal and professional identity. If at all possible, allow the conversation about the spoken word video to evolve organically, directed by the learners' curiosity. After the learners have seen and heard Ms. Bailey's video performance, you may wish to distribute a transcript of Ms. Bailey's spoken word poem. I have found the discussion tends to be richer if learners are able to reference the transcript.

NOTE: **Appendix A** has general guidelines for facilitating a health humanities seminar. **Appendix B** has instruction and discussion prompts specific to this activity for faculty facilitators to use if your learners are not able to initiate a robust discussion.

WRITING AND SHARING

The second activity is for the learner to write to a prompt that directly links the chapter content and the short story. Here is a suggested writing prompt:

You are one of the health professionals who has been taking care of Jasmine. Write a response to Jasmine.

Faculty facilitators can invite the learners to share what they have written with the group. Learners should never be required to share their writings.

REFERENCE LIST

Abreu, B. C. (2006). Professional identity and workplace integration. *American Journal of Occupational Therapy, 60*, 596–599.

American Association of Colleges of Nursing. (n.d.). *About ELNEC*. Retrieved from www.aacnnursing.org/ELNEC/About

Barr, H., Ford, J., Gray, R., Helme, M., Hutchings, M., Low, H., Machin, A., & Reeves, S. (2017). Interprofessional education guidelines 2017. *Centre for the Advancement of Interprofessional Education*. Retrieved from www.caipe.org/resources/publications/caipe-publications/

Bebeau, M. J., & Faber-Langendoen, K. (2014). Remediating lapses in professionalism. In A. Kalet & C. Chou (Eds.), *Remediation in medical education: A mid-course correction* (pp. 103–127). New York: Springer.

Brison, S. J. (2002). *Aftermath: Violence and the remaking of a self*. Princeton, NJ: Princeton University Press.

Cooke, M., Irby, D. M., O'Brien, B. C., & Shulman, L. S. (2010). *Educating physicians: A call for reform of medical school and residency*. San Francisco, CA: Jossey-Bass.

Cruess, R. L., Cruess, S. R., Boudreau, J. D., Snell, L., & Steinert, Y. (2015). A schematic representation of the professional identity formation and socialization of medical students and residents: A guide for medical educators. *Academic Medicine, 90*, 718–725.

Emmanuel, S. M. (Ed.). (2013). *A companion to Buddhist philosophy*. West Sussex, UK: Wiley-Blackwell.

Erikson, E. H. (1964). *Insight and responsibility: Lectures on the ethical implications of psychoanalytic insight*. New York: W. W. Norton & Company.

Erikson, E. H. (1968). *Identity, youth, and crisis*. New York: W. W. Norton & Company.

Hafferty, F. W., & O'Donnell, J. F. (Eds.). (2015). *The hidden curriculum in health professional education*. Hanover, NH: Dartmouth College.

Hammick, M., Freeth, D., Koppel, I., Reeves, S., & Barr, H. (2007). A best evidence systematic review of interprofessional education: BEME Guide no. 9. *Medical Teacher, 29*, 735–751.

Healthy People 2020. (2018). *Determinants of health*. Office of Disease Prevention and Health Promotion. Retrieved from www.healthypeople.gov/2020/about/foundation-health-measures/Determinants-of-Health

Hermans, H. J. M. (2001). The dialogical self: Toward a theory of personal and cultural positioning. *Culture & Psychology, 7*(3), 243–281.

Khalili, H., Orchard, C., Spence Laschinger, H. K., & Farah, R. (2013). An interprofessional socialization framework for developing an interprofessional identity among health professions students. *Journal of Interprofessional Care, 27*(6), 448–453.

Kind, A. (2015). *Persons and personal identity*. Cambridge and Malden, MA: Polity.

Kopf, G. (2015). *Beyond personal identity: Dogen, Nishida, and a phenomenology of no-self*. London and New York: Routledge, Taylor & Francis.

Kornfield, J. (1993). *A path with heart: A guide through the perils and promises of spiritual life*. New York: Bantam.

Le Guin, U. K. (1998). *Lao Tzu: Tao Te Ching: A book about the way and the power of the Way*. Boston, MA and London: Shambhala Publications.

Levine, R. V. (2016). *Stranger in the mirror: The scientific search for self*. Princeton, NJ: Princeton University Press.

Lindemann, H. (2014). *Holding and letting go: The social practice of personal identities*. New York: Oxford University Press.

Locke, J. (1996). *An essay concerning human understanding, 1689*. Abridged and Edited by K. P. Winkler. Indianapolis, IN: Hacket Publishing Company.

Longaker, C. (1997). *Facing death and finding hope: A guide to the emotional and spiritual care of the dying*. New York: Doubleday.

Madell, G. (2015). *The essence of the self: In defense of the simple view of personal identity*. London and New York: Routledge, Taylor & Francis.

McLean, K. C. (2016). *The co-authored self: Family stories and the construction of personal identity*. New York: Oxford University Press.

McNeil, K. A., Mitchell, R. J., & Parker, V. (2013). Interprofessional practice and professional identity threat. *Health Sociology Review, 22*(3), 291–307.

Montenegro, R. E. (2016). My name is not "interpreter." *JAMA, 315*(19), 2071–2072.

Olayiwola, J. N. (2016). Racism in medicine: Shifting the power. *Annals of Family Medicine, 14,* 267–269.

Palmer, P. (2004). *A hidden wholeness: The journey toward an undivided life.* San Francisco, CA: Jossey-Bass.

Palmer, P., & Scribner, M. (2007). *The courage to teach: Guide for reflection and renewal.* San Francisco, CA: Jossey-Bass.

Parfit, D. (1984). *Reasons and persons.* Oxford: Clarendon.

Penuel, W. R., & Wertsch, J. V. (1995). Vygotsky and identity formation: A sociocultural approach. *Educational Psychologist, 30*(2), 83–92.

Quante, M. (2017). *Personal identity as a principle of biomedical ethics.* Cham, CH: Springer International.

Rabow, M. W., Evans, C., & Remen, R. N. (2013). Professional formation and deformation: Repression of personal values and qualities in medical education. *Family Medicine, 45*(1), 13–18.

Sahrmann, S. A. (2014). The human movement system: Our professional identity. *Physical Therapy, 94,* 1034–1042.

Schectman, M. (2014). *Staying alive: Personal identity, practical concerns, and the unity of a life.* New York: Oxford University Press.

Simmons, R. (Producer). (2009). *Brave new voices: Sickle cell by Jasmine Bailey.* HBO. Retrieved from www.youtube.com/watch?v=1OKkzFlWvbA

Sinnott, J. D. (2017). Cognitive underpinnings of identity flexibllity. In J. D. Sinnott (Ed.), *Identity flexibility in adulthood: Perspectives in adult development* (doi:10.1007/978-3-319-55658-1_2). Cham, CH: Springer International.

Sokol, J. T. (2009). Identity development throughout the lifetime: An examination of Eriksonian Theory. *Graduate Journal of Counseling Psychology, 1*(2), article 14. Retrieved from http://epublications.marquette.edu/gjcp/vol1/iss2/14

Ten Hoeve, Y., Jansen, G., & Roodbol, P. (2014). The nursing profession: Public image, self-concept and professional identity. *Journal of Advanced Nursing, 70*(2), 295–309.

Ting-Toomey, S. (2015). Identity negotiation theory. In J. M. Bennett (Ed.), *The Sage encyclopedia of intercultural competence* (doi:10.4135/9781483346267.n143). Thousand Oaks, CA: Sage.

Webb, S. A. (Ed.). (2017). *Professional identity and social work*. Abingdon and New York: Routledge, Taylor & Francis.

APPENDIX A
GENERAL GUIDELINES FOR LEADING A HEALTH HUMANITIES SEMINAR

OVERVIEW

There are many ways to approach health humanities education. I designed the curricular content presented here such that learners have the opportunity to explore questions about the human experience from several perspectives. To paraphrase American journalist, Bill Moyers, the curricular content is intended to nudge learners to question their answers, not answer their questions.

The health humanities curriculum presented in this text is entirely in service to developing clinical skills. The literary and artistic artifacts allow us to hear stories from patients, family members, and healthcare workers without the intensity, time constraint, and competing responsibilities of clinical care. In effect, each artifact that we work with, be it written word, video, audio, or visual art, is the equivalent of a clinical encounter. However, unlike a true clinical encounter, we can go slowly, drill down, revisit parts, question, explore – essentially we can do what we need to improve our understanding of the author's experience, without worrying that we have caused harm. Once we have some perspective on the experience projected by the artifact, we look at our personal reaction to the artifact, as health professionals and simply as human beings. Our personal reactions are a mirror for our deeply held beliefs and biases – some of which serve our performance as health professionals and some of which do not. Once brought to light, these beliefs and biases can be purposefully dismantled and reassembled if need be.

ROLE OF THE FACILITATOR

The most important role of the facilitator is to create a safe, supportive environment for learners to explore and express their feelings about the world of clinical medicine. The facilitator is not present as a content expert, but rather functions as a guide – continually helping learners achieve new levels of self-discovery.

TIPS FOR FACILITATION

The following list of tips derive from conversations I have had over the years with Rita Charon, MD, PhD, Columbia University College of Physicians and Surgeons, Donald Boudreau, MD, McGill University, and Rachel Naomi Remen, MD and Evangeline Andarsio, MD, Remen Institute for the Study of Health and Illness.

1 **Remember, there is nothing to teach.** As a facilitator, your focus is not on teaching content, but rather on providing opportunity for, and guiding learners toward, self-exploration and discovery. Each learner will participate in his or her own way.

2 **Avoid the temptation to interpret the learners' written and verbal expression**.
   You can probe and/or highlight features (e.g., shifting pronouns, evocative words)
   as a means of helping the learner interpret his or her own expression; however,
   interpretation from you, as a health professions educator, may feel threatening to
   the learner and inappropriately carry a diagnostic authority. Remember, this is not
   group therapy.

3 **(Mostly) avoid bringing your own story into the room.** You likely have a wealth
   of personal and professional stories that undoubtedly form a wellspring of wisdom
   for the learners. The health humanities seminars, however, are probably not the
   time to share those stories. It is far too easy for learners to dodge the hard work
   of self-reflection by relying on your stories for insight. This is the learners' time to
   have their *own* insights. That said, there may be times when sharing your story will
   encourage learners to dig deeper into their own experience. Sharing your story can
   also reduce perceived hierarchy in the group and add to group cohesion. Use your
   judgment as to when it is appropriate to bring your story into the room.

4 **Allow the themes for the sessions to arise organically.** Although I provide
   learning objectives for each session, I encourage you to allow themes for the
   sessions to arise organically from the reading, writing, and discussion. As with all
   experiential learning activities, outcomes from the health humanities seminars will
   often not be fully and immediately apparent to you or the learners. Think of the
   seminar as planting seeds in fertile soil – you are not entirely sure what will take
   root, what will flourish, and what will lay dormant for a season or two.

5 **Learners should do most of the talking in the seminars.** Your job is to lob
   questions into the conversation to help the learners have a more sophisticated
   experience with the material and with each other.

EMOTIONALLY EVOCATIVE ACTIVITIES

The activities may be emotionally evocative for learners. Discussion and writing prompts
may lead learners to express their personal experience with illness or caring for an ill
family member. Learners may also share attitudes, beliefs, and values from their religious
or cultural group. These stories, while richly human and educational, also have the
potential to be emotionally evocative – which in turn can be uncomfortable for learners
who are not accustomed to exploring emotions. Here are two ways to honor the story and
the emotion, while taking the group's attention off the emotionally wrought learner.

1 To the learner: "Thank you for sharing your story. Your experience will help you
   become an attentive health professional."
   To the group: "Can anyone suggest how [Learner X's] experience will add to [his/
   her] clinical skills?" You can encourage answers such as: compassion, empathy,
   understanding, attention to detail, observations skills, whatever else you deem
   appropriate to the story.

2 To the learner: "Thank you for sharing your story."

To the group: "Has anyone else experienced something like this?" If someone volunteers, you can invite that person to share his or her story. If no one volunteers, you can say, "At some point, all of us will have an experience like [Learner X]. It is part of being a human. And while it's a sad story, you can see how that story will motivate [Learner X] to help many other people as a health professional."

EMOTIONAL DISTANCING

Please keep in mind that some of our learners may need to emotionally distance themselves from the activities, especially if they have personal experience with the illness, injury, or topic at hand. Emotional distancing is commonly expressed as humor, derision, and/or fixating on the biomedical elements of the story. The potential exists for a "teachable moment" if you *gently* highlight the behavior as emotional distancing while not making the learner feel exposed or antagonized.

ADDITIONAL RESOURCES FOR FACILITATORS

Facilitating a health humanities seminar is unlike other educational activities. Prior to meeting with learners, facilitators should seek training and mentorship from faculty who are experienced leading health humanities seminars. The following resources may be helpful to orient new facilitators and refresh the skills of mature facilitators.

Charon, R., Das Gupta, S., Hermann, N., Irvine, C., Marcus, E. R., Rivera Colon, E., Spencer, D., & Spiegel, M. (2017). *The principles and practices of narrative medicine.* New York: Oxford University Press.

Miller, A., Grohe, M., Shahram, K., & Katz, J. T. (2013). From the galleries to the clinic: Applying art museum lessons to patient care. *Journal of Medical Humanities, 34*(3). doi:10.1007/s10912-013-9250-8.

APPENDIX B
DISCUSSION PROMPTS

CHAPTER 2 LEARNER ACTIVITY ESSAY,
DESPERATELY SEEKING HERB WEINMAN

What do we know about Mr. Lewis? Read aloud places in the text that give you this impression.

What are Mr. Lewis's perceptions of the health professionals who care for him? Do you think his perceptions are unique to his experience or typical of other patients?

In what ways could Mr. Lewis's expectations of healthcare professionals influence his illness experience?

What do you think Mr. Lewis's illness narrative is?

What do you think the health professionals in this story have as an illness narrative?

CHAPTER 3 LEARNER ACTIVITY VIDEO,
REBECCA BERKOWITZ: MY QUIT SMOKING STORY

NOTE

Having read chapter 3 Unconscious Bias, some learners may be disinclined to reveal their biases to the group. As you know from personal experience, it takes a great deal of courage and vulnerability to recognize and reveal our unconscious mind to ourselves and to others. I encourage you to acknowledge the learners' efforts at reflection and self-awareness.

As facilitator, you must decide what level of discourse is appropriate for your group. Personally, I state early in the session that it can be uncomfortable to confront our biases, but once we do, it can feel liberating. Confrontation is the first step toward mitigation. You must predict what will work best for your group based on your knowledge of the group dynamic. This might be a session where talking about your own biases in the clinical setting could be helpful for the learners. Please use your judgment about what you are willing to disclose and whether your group is ready to hear it.

I deliberately chose the unconscious bias artifact to relate to a person who smokes. For most of us, it is easier to admit bias against a smoker than against a racial, ethnic, religious group, or sexual minority. Ms. Berkowitz may trigger unconscious biases beyond her smoker status such as her characteristics as an older woman who is overweight.

PROMPTS

Ms. Berkowitz says, "I will be non-smoker – believe it or not." Do you believe her? Why or why not?

What do you think about the way Ms. Berkowitz talked about her relationship with her doctor?

Did your opinion of Ms. Berkowitz stay the same throughout the video or did your opinion change? If it changed, what did Ms. Berkowitz say or do to make your opinion change?

Did Ms. Berkowitz's piano performance influence your assessment of her ability to quit smoking?

CHAPTER 4 LEARNER ACTIVITY PODCAST, *FALLING SLOWLY*

What is your experience of bearing witness to Lee-anna's story?

What emotions are conveyed at the beginning of the story?

What emotional shifts do you notice as the story progresses?

What parts of Lee-anna's story surprised you?

Did you have a reaction to Lee-anna's description of falling? [You may wish to point out that highly focused attention and suspension of time are common features among trauma stories, regardless of the type of trauma (motor vehicle crash, violent attack, sports injury, etc.).]

Do any parts of Lee-anna's story relate to your clinical experiences?

CHAPTER 5 LEARNER ACTIVITY PHOTOGALLERY, *THE SCAR PROJECT*

NOTE

To lead a comprehensive investigation of *The Scar Project* photographs, you will need to develop skills using Visual Thinking Strategies (VTS). VTS is a teaching methodology that helps learners look carefully and attentively, interpret what they are seeing, communicate the evidence for their interpretations, and participate in respectful discourse about alternative interpretations and meaning (Yenawine, 2013). For discussion about applying Visual Thinking Strategies in health professional education, see the article, *From the Galleries to the Clinic: Applying Art Museum Lessons to Patient Care* (Miller, Grohe, Shahram, & Katz, 2013).

PROMPTS

The standard VTS questions are 1) What's going on in the image? 2) What do you see that makes you say that? 3) What more can you see?

Do you see evidence of resilience? Show us where.

Why is it difficult to look?

What do you think would motivate a woman to participate in this project?

When people come to view the exhibit in a museum, what do you think they're looking for (or hoping to see)?

CHAPTER 6 LEARNER ACTIVITY BOOK EXCERPT, *BRIGHT HOUR*

Who is in relationship with whom in this story? Whoever is mentioned, ask all the learners to look in the text for an indicator of the relationship and the nature of the relationship – and then to read that section aloud.

Why do you think Dr. Cavanaugh told Nina about the time she counseled her son about inviting a girl to a dance?

What emotions are conveyed in the story? Whatever emotion the learner mentions, ask all the learners to look in the text for examples of that emotion, and then read that section aloud.

Dr. Cavanaugh says to Nina, "I just want you to know that I still feel like we're in a good place on this." Why do you think she said "... we're in a good place ..." and not "... *you're* in a good place ..."?

Do any parts of the story relate to chapter 6 or to your clinical experiences?

CHAPTER 7 LEARNER ACTIVITY SHORT STORY, *QUILL*

What emotions are conveyed in the story? Whatever emotion is mentioned, ask all the learners to look in the text for examples of that emotion, and then read that section aloud.

Invite the learners to identify passages where the characters are expressing: *admiration, ambivalence, kindness, forgiveness, fear, regret*. Note for the learners that these words are never used in the story and yet they are able to recognize the emotions – these are examples of subtext.

What are the relationships in this story? Whoever is mentioned, ask all the learners to look in the text for an indicator of the relationship and the nature of the relationship – and then to read that section aloud. You can guide the learners to consider the relationships between:

Present day Quill and Thompson;

Childhood Quill and Thompson;

Present day Quill and Childhood Thompson;

Present day Thompson and Childhood Quill;

Quill and his inner self (both as an adult and as a child);

Thompson and his inner self (both as an adult and as a child).

What aspects of the brothers' relationship change over time in the story? What aspects of the brothers' relationship endure over time?

Do any parts of the story relate to chapter 7 or to your clinical experiences?

CHAPTER 8 LEARNER ACTIVITY POEM, *TUBES*

What do you hear in the line, "Grief weighs down the seesaw; joy cannot budge it"?

What do you hear in the line, "We were always," he said glancing down, "a fool two years ago"?

Why do you think the author repeatedly describes the character as. . . "The man with the tubes up his nose [nostrils]"?

How do you think "the man with the tubes up his nose" feels about his treatment decisions? What lines in the poem support your supposition?

Do any parts of the story relate to your clinical experiences? Whatever is mentioned, ask all the learners to look in the text for examples and then read that section aloud.

CHAPTER 9 LEARNER ACTIVITY SPOKEN WORD VIDEO, *SICKLE CELL*

NOTE

When learners write in the role of the health professional, some may be inclined toward feelings of guilt or shame at having hurt Jasmine, while others may feel indignant that

Jasmine is unappreciative of their efforts to help. Regardless of the feelings expressed by the learners, the facilitator's responsibility is to guide the learners to understand that Jasmine is expressing *her perspective* on sickle cell disease. While health professionals likely have a different perspective on the disease, it is still possible to honor and value the patient's perspective without being self-recriminatory or defensive.

PROMPTS

Who is Jasmine talking to?

What do you think contributes to Jasmine's personal identity? Where in the poem do you find support for your supposition?

Do you think Jasmine feels that her personal identity is recognized by her health professionals or her peers? Where in the poem do you find support for your supposition?

What emotions does Jasmine convey in the piece? Whatever emotion is mentioned, ask all the learners to look in the text for examples of that emotion, and then read that section aloud.

Do any parts of the story relate to chapter 9 or your clinical experiences?

REFERENCE LIST

Miller, A., Grohe, M., Shahram, K., & Katz, J. T. (2013). From the galleries to the clinic: Applying art museum lessons to patient care. *Journal of Medical Humanities, 34*(3). doi:10.1007/s10912-013-9250-8

Yenawine, P. (2013). *Visual thinking strategies: Using art to deepen learning across school disciplines.* Cambridge, MA: Harvard Education.

INDEX

Note: Page numbers in *italics* indicate a figure, and page numbers in **bold** indicate a table on the corresponding page.